Building The Perfect Body

The Definitive Manual On Scientific Methods For Increasing Muscle Mass, Reducing Body Fat, And Enhancing Physical Performance

BY MR JOE

Table of Contents

Introduction

Welcome to "Building the Perfect Body: The Definitive Manual on Scientific Methods for Increasing Muscle Mass, Reducing Body Fat, and Enhancing Physical Performance." This ebook is designed to be your ultimate guide in the journey toward achieving your ideal physique. Whether you're a complete beginner or a seasoned fitness enthusiast, this book will provide you with the knowledge and tools to transform your body and improve your overall health.

In today's world, we're bombarded with countless fitness fads, miracle diets, and quick-fix solutions. It's easy to feel overwhelmed and confused about what really works. This book cuts through the noise by presenting scientifically-backed methods that have been proven to yield results. By following the advice and strategies outlined here, you'll be able to build muscle, lose fat, and enhance your physical performance in a sustainable and effective way.

Target Audience

This book is tailored for men and women between the ages of 18 and 45 living in the United States. Whether you're a college student looking to get fit, a young professional trying to balance work and health, or a parent wanting to set a good example for your kids, this book is for you. We've considered the unique challenges and opportunities faced by American youth, ensuring the advice is relevant and applicable to your lifestyle.

How to Use This Book

Before diving into the chapters, it's important to understand how to make the most out of this ebook. Here's a quick guide:

Start at the Beginning: The foundational concepts in Part I are crucial for understanding the more advanced strategies discussed later. Don't skip these sections, even if you're eager to jump into the workouts or nutrition plans.

Apply What You Learn: Knowledge without action is useless. Each chapter includes practical tips and actionable steps. Make sure to implement these in your daily routine.

Track Your Progress: Keep a journal or use a fitness app to record your workouts, meals, and progress. This will help you stay accountable and make necessary adjustments.

Stay Flexible: Everyone's body responds differently to various stimuli. Be prepared to tweak your plan based on your individual needs and progress.

Seek Support: Share your goals with friends, family, or a fitness community. Having a support system can keep you motivated and on track.

The Importance of a Scientific Approach

One of the core principles of this book is the reliance on science. In an era where misinformation is rampant, especially in the fitness industry, it's crucial to base your approach on reliable, evidence-based information. Here's why:

Consistency Over Fads: Scientific methods have stood the test of time and rigorous testing. Unlike fad diets and trendy workouts that come and go, a scientific approach provides consistency and reliability.

Personalization: Understanding the science behind fitness allows you to tailor your program to your unique needs. What works for one person might not work for another, and a scientific approach helps you find what works best for you.

Safety: Many quick-fix solutions can be harmful or unsustainable. By following scientifically-backed methods, you reduce the risk of injury and ensure your efforts are safe and effective.

Sustainability: Achieving your fitness goals is not about temporary fixes but about long-term lifestyle changes. Science-based strategies are designed to be sustainable, helping you maintain your progress over the long haul.

In the following chapters, we will delve into the science of muscle growth, fat loss, and performance enhancement. We'll debunk common myths, provide you with actionable advice, and equip you with the knowledge to make informed decisions about your fitness journey.

Get ready to embark on a transformative journey. With dedication, patience, and the right knowledge, you can build the perfect body. Let's get started!

Part I: The Foundations of Fitness

Chapter 1: The Science of Muscle Growth

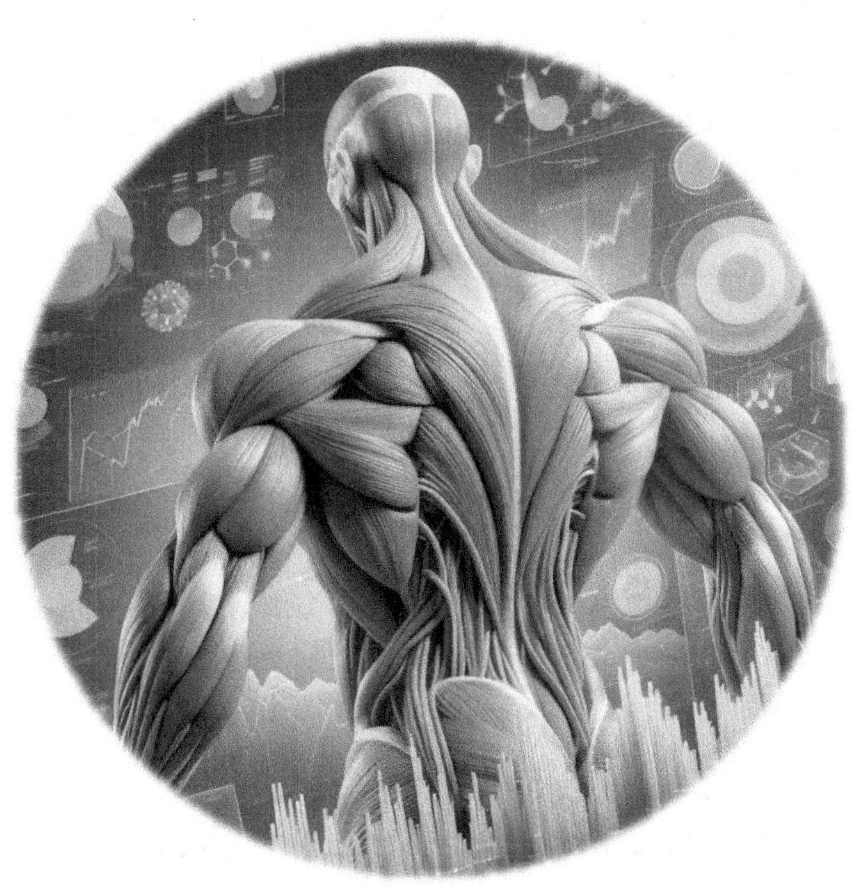

Understanding Muscle Anatomy

To understand how to build muscle effectively, it's essential to start with the basics of muscle anatomy. Knowing how your muscles are structured and function can provide invaluable insight into the best ways to stimulate growth and achieve your fitness goals.

Muscle Structure

Your muscles are made up of bundles of muscle fibers, which are, in turn, composed of smaller units called myofibrils. Each muscle fiber is a single cell that can contract and produce force. When you lift weights or perform resistance training, you're essentially challenging these muscle fibers, causing them to adapt and grow stronger.

Here's a simple breakdown of the key components of muscle anatomy:

Muscle Fibers: These are the basic building blocks of muscles. Muscle fibers come in different types, each with unique properties and functions.

Myofibrils: These are tiny strands within each muscle fiber. Myofibrils contain the contractile proteins actin and myosin, which interact to produce muscle contractions.

Fascicles: Bundles of muscle fibers are grouped together into fascicles. Each fascicle is surrounded by connective tissue called perimysium.

Epimysium and Endomysium: The entire muscle is encased in a layer of connective tissue called the epimysium, while each individual muscle fiber is surrounded by the endomysium.

Understanding this structure is crucial because it helps explain how muscles grow and adapt to resistance training. When you lift weights, you create tiny tears in the muscle fibers. These microtears are a good thing – they signal your body to repair the damage and, in the process, make the muscle stronger and larger.

Types of Muscle Fibers

Not all muscle fibers are created equal. There are two primary types of muscle fibers, each with different characteristics:

Type I (Slow-Twitch) Fibers: These fibers are more endurance-oriented and are great for activities like long-distance running or cycling. They contract slowly and can sustain activity for longer periods without fatigue.

Type II (Fast-Twitch) Fibers: These fibers are more power-oriented and are used for short bursts of intense activity, like sprinting or lifting heavy weights. They contract quickly and generate a lot of force but fatigue more rapidly.

Most people have a mix of both fiber types, but the ratio can vary based on genetics and training history. Understanding your muscle fiber composition can help you tailor your training to maximize growth and performance. For instance, if you have a higher proportion of fast-twitch fibers, you might respond better to heavy lifting and explosive movements.

The Role of Satellite Cells

Satellite cells are a type of stem cell found in muscles that play a crucial role in muscle repair and growth. When you exercise, especially during resistance training, satellite cells are activated. They then multiply and fuse with damaged muscle fibers, helping to repair and rebuild them. This process not only repairs the muscle but also adds new nuclei to the muscle cells, enhancing their capacity for growth.

The Neuromuscular Connection

Another key component of muscle anatomy is the neuromuscular junction – the point where nerve cells meet muscle fibers. When you decide to lift a weight, your brain sends a signal through your nervous system to the relevant muscles. This signal reaches the neuromuscular junction, releasing a chemical called acetylcholine, which triggers muscle contraction.

This neuromuscular connection is vital for muscle growth because it determines how effectively your muscles can contract and produce force. Regular resistance training can enhance this connection, making your muscles more efficient and responsive.

Hypertrophy: How Muscles Grow

Muscle hypertrophy is the technical term for muscle growth. There are two main types of hypertrophy:

Sarcoplasmic Hypertrophy: This type of growth involves an increase in the volume of the sarcoplasm, the fluid within muscle cells. It's typically associated with higher-repetition, lower-weight training and can increase muscle size without significantly boosting strength.

Myofibrillar Hypertrophy: This involves an increase in the number and size of myofibrils within muscle fibers. It's typically associated with lower-repetition, higher-weight training and leads to both increased muscle size and strength.

Both types of hypertrophy are important for overall muscle development, and a balanced training program should include elements that promote each type.

Practical Tips for Stimulating Muscle Growth

Now that you have a solid understanding of muscle anatomy and how muscles grow, let's look at some practical tips for stimulating muscle growth:

Progressive Overload: Continuously challenging your muscles by gradually increasing the weight, reps, or intensity of your workouts is key to promoting muscle growth.

Varied Training: Incorporate different types of exercises and training modalities to target all muscle fibers and prevent adaptation.

Adequate Nutrition: Ensure you're consuming enough protein to support muscle repair and growth. Aim for a balanced diet that includes all essential nutrients.

Rest and Recovery: Muscles grow during rest, not during the workout itself. Ensure you're getting enough sleep and allowing adequate recovery time between workouts.

Consistency: Consistent training over time is essential for long-term muscle growth. Stay committed and patient.

By understanding the science behind muscle growth and applying these principles, you'll be well on your way to building a stronger, more muscular physique. The next chapters will delve deeper into specific strategies and techniques to help you achieve your fitness goals.

Mechanisms Of Muscle Hypertrophy

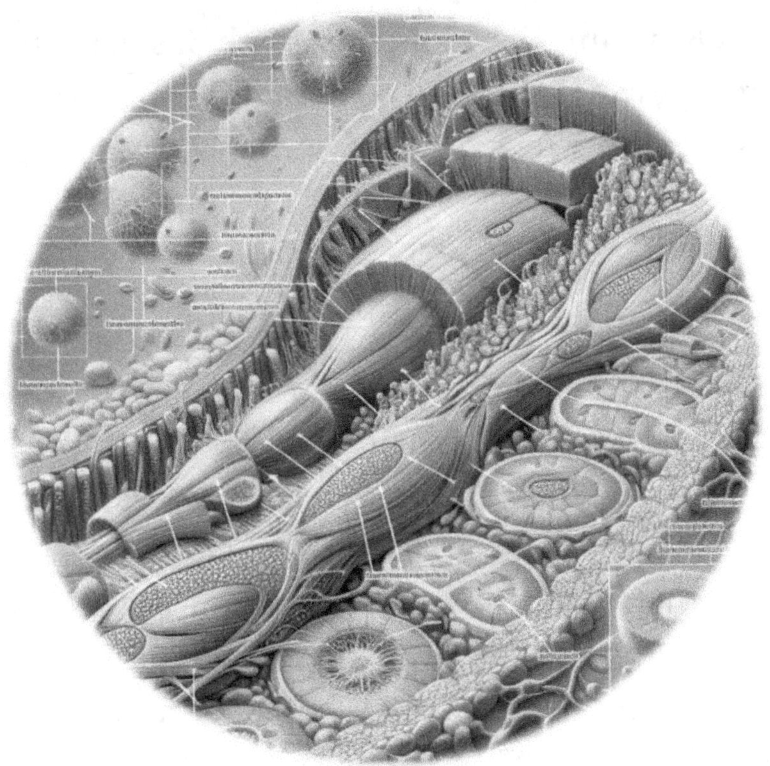

Understanding the mechanisms behind muscle hypertrophy is essential for anyone serious about building muscle. Muscle hypertrophy refers to the increase in muscle size and is primarily driven by three key factors: mechanical tension, muscle damage, and metabolic stress. Let's dive into each of these mechanisms and how they contribute to muscle growth.

Mechanical Tension

Mechanical tension is one of the most critical factors for muscle hypertrophy. It occurs when muscles generate force against resistance. This tension creates stress on the muscle fibers, signaling the body to adapt and grow stronger. Here's how it works:

Tension Over Time: For muscle growth, it's not just about lifting heavy weights but also about how long the muscles are under tension. This is where the concept of "time under tension" (TUT) comes into play. By controlling the tempo of your lifts, you can increase TUT and maximize muscle activation.

Progressive Overload: Continuously increasing the weight or resistance you use in your workouts forces your muscles to adapt to new levels of stress. This principle, known as progressive overload, is fundamental to long-term muscle growth. For example, if you bench press 150 pounds today, aim to lift 155 pounds next week. Small, incremental increases add up over time, pushing your muscles to grow.

Muscle Damage

When you engage in resistance training, especially with new or intense exercises, you cause tiny tears in your muscle fibers. This muscle damage is not harmful; in fact, it's a crucial part of the muscle growth process. The body responds to these microtears by repairing the damaged fibers, making them thicker and stronger than before. Here's a closer look at how muscle damage contributes to hypertrophy:

Eccentric Training: The eccentric phase of a lift, where the muscle lengthens under tension (like lowering the barbell in a bench press), causes more muscle damage than the concentric phase (lifting the barbell). Incorporating eccentric-focused exercises can enhance muscle growth. For example, try slowing down the lowering phase of your lifts to increase muscle damage.

Variety in Exercises: Constantly challenging your muscles with new exercises can lead to more muscle damage and growth. This is why varying your workout routine every few weeks is beneficial. For instance, if you usually perform squats, try adding lunges or leg presses to your routine.

Metabolic Stress

Metabolic stress, often referred to as "the pump," is the burning sensation you feel in your muscles during high-rep, high-intensity workouts. This stress occurs due to the accumulation of metabolites like lactate, hydrogen ions, and inorganic phosphates. While metabolic stress alone won't build muscle, it plays a significant role in hypertrophy. Here's how:

Cell Swelling: The accumulation of metabolites causes cells to swell, triggering a response that leads to muscle growth. This phenomenon is known as "cellular swelling" or "the pump." It creates an environment that promotes protein synthesis and muscle growth.

High-Rep Training: Incorporating high-rep sets (15-20 reps) into your routine can increase metabolic stress. For example, after your heavy sets of squats, try doing a few sets of lighter, high-rep leg extensions to achieve a good pump.

Hormonal Response

Exercise, especially resistance training, triggers the release of hormones that facilitate muscle growth. The most notable hormone in this process is testosterone, which plays a crucial role in protein synthesis and muscle repair. Additionally, growth hormone and insulin-like growth factor (IGF-1) are also important for muscle hypertrophy. Here's how hormones contribute to muscle growth:

Testosterone Boost: Compound exercises like squats, deadlifts, and bench presses stimulate a significant testosterone response. Including these exercises in your routine can enhance muscle growth. For example, performing a heavy set of deadlifts can boost your testosterone levels more effectively than isolation exercises.

Growth Hormone Release: Intense training and short rest periods can increase the release of growth hormone. Incorporating techniques like high-intensity interval training (HIIT) or circuit training can maximize this effect.

Protein Synthesis and Breakdown

Muscle hypertrophy occurs when protein synthesis (building new proteins) exceeds protein breakdown (the natural degradation of proteins). Resistance training stimulates protein synthesis, while adequate nutrition, particularly protein intake, supports this process. Here's how to optimize protein synthesis:

Post-Workout Nutrition: Consuming protein after your workout helps kickstart the muscle repair and growth process. Aim for 20-30 grams of high-quality protein within an hour of finishing your workout. For example, a protein shake or a meal with lean meat, fish, or eggs can be effective.

Consistent Protein Intake: Spread your protein intake throughout the day to maintain a positive protein balance. Aim for 1.2 to 2.2 grams of protein per kilogram of body weight per day, depending on your training intensity and goals. For instance, if you weigh 70 kilograms (154 pounds), aim for at least 84 grams of protein daily.

Practical Tips for Maximizing Muscle Hypertrophy

To effectively apply the principles of muscle hypertrophy, consider these practical tips:

Combine Training Styles: Use a mix of heavy, low-rep sets and lighter, high-rep sets to target all aspects of muscle growth. For example, start with heavy squats for 4-6 reps, followed by leg presses for 12-15 reps.

Focus on Form: Proper form ensures you're effectively targeting the intended muscles and reduces the risk of injury. For instance, when performing a bench press, ensure your shoulder blades are retracted and your elbows are at a 45-degree angle to your body.

Incorporate Compound Movements: Exercises that engage multiple muscle groups, like deadlifts, bench presses, and pull-ups, create more mechanical tension and hormonal response. Include these movements regularly in your routine.

Utilize Periodization: Periodization involves cycling through different phases of training, such as hypertrophy, strength, and endurance phases. This approach helps prevent plateaus and promotes continuous progress.

Prioritize Recovery: Adequate sleep, nutrition, and rest days are essential for muscle repair and growth. Ensure you're getting 7-9 hours of sleep per night and incorporating rest days into your training schedule.

By understanding and applying these mechanisms of muscle hypertrophy, you can create an effective training program that maximizes muscle growth and helps you achieve your fitness goals. In the next chapters, we'll explore specific strategies and techniques to further enhance your muscle-building journey.

The Importance Of Progressive Overload

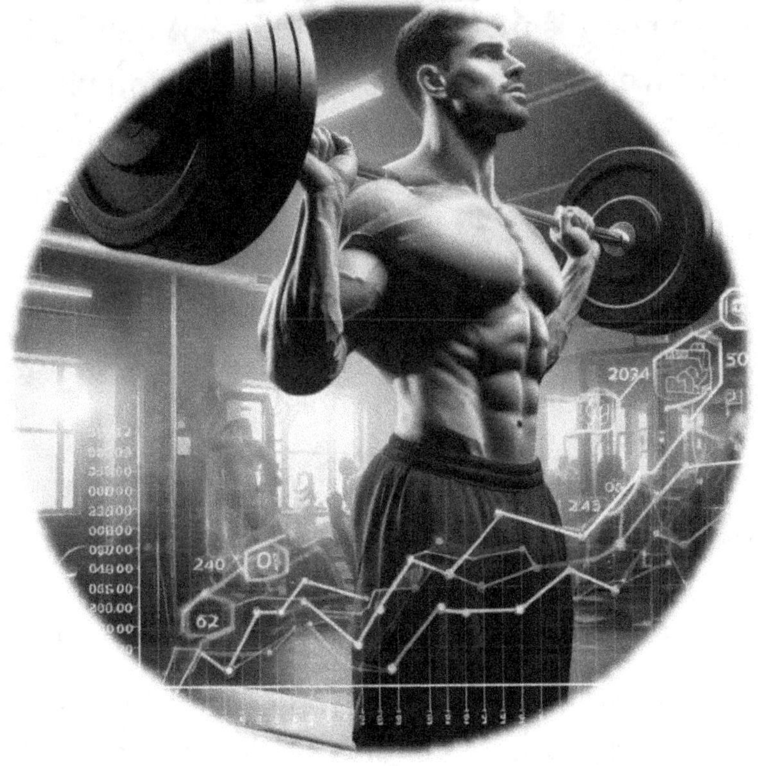

If you've spent any time in the gym, you've likely heard the term "progressive overload." This concept is the backbone of effective muscle growth. In simple terms, progressive overload is the gradual increase of stress placed on the body during exercise. This stress can come from lifting heavier weights, increasing the number of reps, or changing up your workout routine. Understanding and implementing progressive overload is crucial for anyone looking to build muscle, lose fat, and enhance physical performance.

Why Progressive Overload Matters

The human body is incredibly adaptive. When you first start lifting weights, your muscles respond quickly to the new stress, leading to rapid gains in strength and size. However, as your body adapts to the workload, these gains can slow down or even plateau. This is where progressive overload comes in. By continually challenging your muscles with increased stress, you force them to adapt, grow, and become stronger.

Think of your muscles like a team of construction workers. If the workload remains the same, the workers become efficient and complete the job without much effort. But if you gradually increase the workload, the workers must adapt, bring in more resources, and work harder. Similarly, progressively overloading your muscles requires them to recruit more fibers, grow stronger, and increase in size.

Methods of Implementing Progressive Overload

There are several effective ways to incorporate progressive overload into your training routine. Here are some strategies to consider:

Increase the Weight: This is the most straightforward method. By lifting heavier weights, you increase the stress on your muscles. For example, if you bench press 100 pounds for 8 reps, try increasing the weight to 105 pounds the next time. Even small increments can make a big difference over time.

Increase the Reps: Adding more repetitions to your sets can also enhance muscle growth. If you're currently doing 3 sets of 10 reps, try increasing to 12 reps. This increases the volume and overall workload on your muscles.

Increase the Sets: Adding more sets to your routine can also boost progressive overload. If you're performing 3 sets of an exercise, try increasing to 4 or 5 sets. This additional volume can stimulate further muscle growth.

Change the Tempo: Slowing down the eccentric (lowering) phase of an exercise can increase time under tension and stress on the muscles. For example, take 3-4 seconds to lower the weight during a bicep curl, and then lift it back up in 1-2 seconds.

Decrease Rest Time: Reducing the rest time between sets can increase the intensity of your workout. If you typically rest for 90 seconds between sets, try reducing it to 60 seconds. This keeps your muscles under constant stress and can promote growth.

Change Exercises: Introducing new exercises can challenge your muscles in different ways. If you've been doing barbell squats, try switching to front squats or lunges. New movements can target different muscle fibers and stimulate growth.

Examples of Progressive Overload in Action

To illustrate how progressive overload works, let's look at a few examples:

Bench Press: Let's say you currently bench press 150 pounds for 8 reps. Over the next few weeks, you can implement progressive overload by gradually increasing the weight. In week 1, try 155 pounds for 8 reps. In week 2, increase to 160 pounds for 8 reps. By week 4, you might be lifting 170 pounds for 8 reps. This steady increase in weight forces your chest, shoulders, and triceps to adapt and grow stronger.

Squats: If you're doing squats with 200 pounds for 3 sets of 10 reps, you can apply progressive overload by adding more reps. In week 1, try 12 reps per set with the same weight. In week 2, increase to 15 reps per set. Alternatively, you could add another set, doing 4 sets of 10 reps instead of 3. Both strategies increase the workload on your legs, promoting muscle growth.

Bicep Curls: For bicep curls, if you're lifting 25 pounds for 3 sets of 12 reps, try changing the tempo. In week 1, take 3 seconds to lower the weight and 1 second to lift it. In week 2, decrease the rest time between sets from 60 seconds to 45 seconds. These changes increase the intensity and stress on your biceps, encouraging growth.

Tracking Progress

To effectively implement progressive overload, it's essential to track your progress. Keeping a workout log or using a fitness app can help you monitor the weights, reps, and sets you perform. This allows you to see your progress over time and make necessary adjustments to your routine. For example, if you notice that you've been lifting the same weight for several weeks without increasing, it might be time to push yourself and add more weight or reps.

Here's a simple way to track your progress:

Workout Log: Write down the exercises you perform, the weights you use, and the number of sets and reps you complete. Note any changes you make to the tempo or rest time. Review your log regularly to ensure you're consistently increasing the workload.

Fitness Apps: There are many fitness apps available that can help you track your progress. These apps often include features like workout tracking, progress charts, and reminders to help you stay on track.

Overcoming Plateaus

Even with progressive overload, you may hit plateaus where your progress stalls. This is normal and can be overcome with a few strategies:

Deload Weeks: Incorporate a lighter week of training every 4-6 weeks. This allows your muscles to recover and adapt, preventing overtraining and promoting long-term growth.

Variety in Training: Change up your exercises, sets, reps, and rest times regularly. This prevents your body from adapting to a specific routine and keeps your muscles challenged.

Focus on Weak Points: Identify areas where you're struggling and focus on them. If your bench press isn't improving, try adding accessory exercises like tricep dips or chest flies to strengthen supporting muscles.

Practical Tips for Effective Progressive Overload

Be Patient: Progress takes time. Don't rush the process or increase the weight too quickly. Gradual, consistent increases are more sustainable and safer.

Listen to Your Body: Pay attention to how your body responds to increased stress. If you feel pain (not to be confused with the normal discomfort of a tough workout), take a step back and reassess your approach.

Stay Consistent: Consistency is key to long-term success. Stick to your workout plan and make incremental adjustments as needed.

Seek Support: Working with a personal trainer or joining a fitness community can provide additional motivation and guidance.

By understanding and applying the principles of progressive overload, you'll be well-equipped to achieve your muscle growth goals. This concept is a cornerstone of effective training and, when implemented correctly, can lead to significant gains in strength, size, and overall performance. In the following chapters, we'll explore more advanced techniques and strategies to further enhance your muscle-building journey.

Chapter 2: The Physiology Of Fat Loss

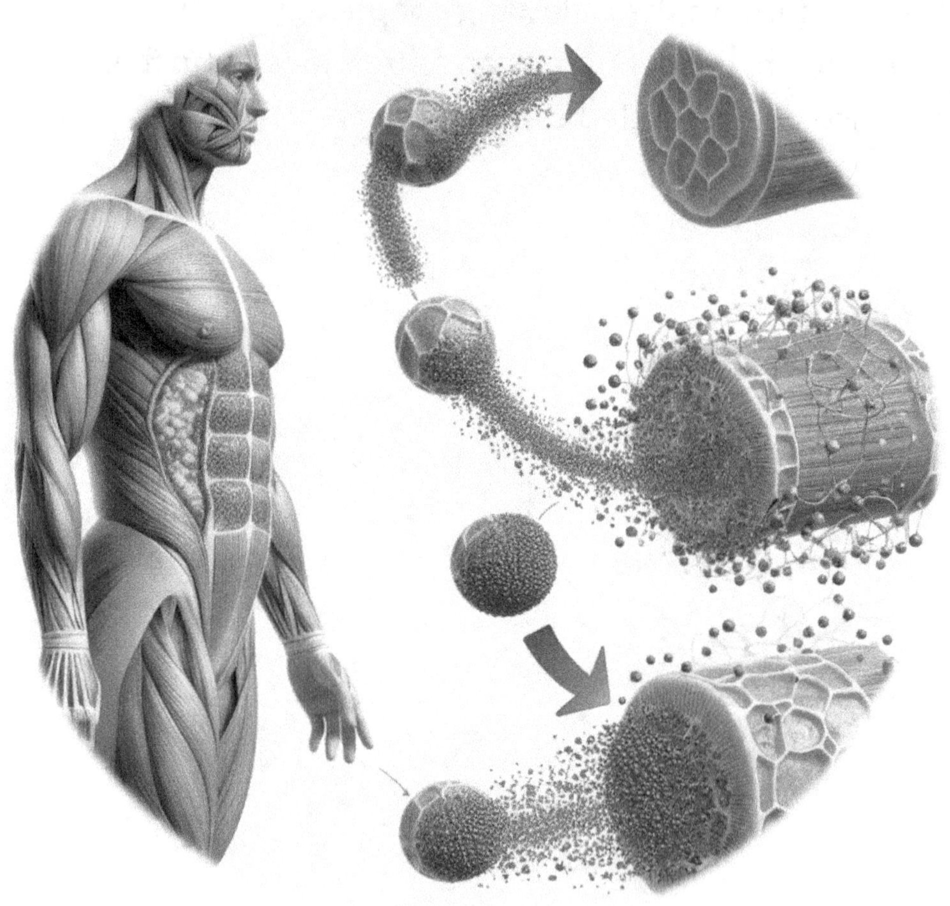

How The Body Stores And Burns Fat

Understanding how your body stores and burns fat is essential for effective fat loss. Fat, or adipose tissue, serves various critical functions in the body, including energy storage, insulation, and protection of vital organs. However, excess fat, particularly visceral fat around the organs, can pose health risks. This chapter will delve into the physiological processes of fat storage and burning, providing a comprehensive understanding of how to effectively manage body fat.

How the Body Stores Fat

When you consume more calories than your body needs for energy, the excess calories are converted into fat and stored in adipose tissue. This process involves several key steps:

Digestion and Absorption: The journey of fat storage begins with the digestion of food. Carbohydrates, proteins, and fats are broken down into their basic components—glucose, amino acids, and fatty acids, respectively—during digestion. These components are then absorbed into the bloodstream.

Insulin's Role: After eating, the pancreas releases insulin, a hormone that helps regulate blood sugar levels. Insulin facilitates the uptake of glucose into cells, where it can be used for energy. When glycogen stores (stored glucose) in the liver and muscles are full, any excess glucose is converted into fatty acids.

Fat Storage: The liver converts excess glucose into fatty acids through a process called de novo lipogenesis. These fatty acids are then packaged into triglycerides and transported to adipose tissue for storage. Adipose tissue, which consists of fat cells called adipocytes, can expand to accommodate increasing amounts of stored fat.

Types of Body Fat

Understanding the different types of body fat can provide insight into how fat is stored and its impact on health:

Subcutaneous Fat: This is the fat stored just beneath the skin. It's the most visible type of fat and can be found in areas like the abdomen, thighs, and arms. While subcutaneous fat is generally less harmful than other types, excess amounts can still contribute to health issues.

Visceral Fat: This fat is stored around internal organs in the abdominal cavity. Visceral fat is more metabolically active and is linked to higher risks of conditions like heart disease, type 2 diabetes, and inflammation. Reducing visceral fat is crucial for improving overall health.

Brown Fat: Unlike white fat (subcutaneous and visceral), brown fat burns energy to produce heat. It's more prevalent in infants but also present in small amounts in adults. Brown fat activation is a topic of interest for fat loss research, as it can potentially aid in burning calories.

How the Body Burns Fat

Burning fat, or lipolysis, is the process of breaking down stored triglycerides into fatty acids and glycerol, which can then be used for energy. Several physiological mechanisms and conditions influence fat burning:

Hormonal Regulation: Hormones play a pivotal role in regulating fat metabolism. Key hormones involved in fat burning include:

Epinephrine and Norepinephrine: These hormones, released during stress or exercise, activate fat breakdown. They bind to receptors on fat cells, triggering the release of stored fatty acids into the bloodstream.

Insulin: While insulin promotes fat storage, low insulin levels (such as during fasting or low-carb diets) facilitate fat burning. Keeping insulin levels stable through diet can enhance fat metabolism.

Glucagon: This hormone, released when blood sugar levels are low, stimulates the release of stored fat for energy.

Energy Expenditure: Your body requires a certain amount of energy (calories) to maintain basic functions like breathing, circulation, and cell production—this is known as the basal metabolic rate (BMR). Physical activity, from walking to high-intensity exercise, increases your total energy expenditure (TEE), prompting your body to use stored fat for fuel.

Lipolysis and Fat Oxidation: During lipolysis, triglycerides stored in fat cells are broken down into free fatty acids and glycerol. These fatty acids are then transported to mitochondria, the energy-producing structures within cells, where they undergo oxidation to produce ATP (adenosine triphosphate), the primary energy currency of the body.

Factors Influencing Fat Storage and Burning

Several factors influence how efficiently your body stores and burns fat:

Genetics: Genetic makeup can affect fat distribution, metabolic rate, and how easily you gain or lose weight. While you can't change your genetics, understanding your predispositions can help tailor your fat loss strategies.

Diet: The types and amounts of food you eat significantly impact fat storage and burning. Diets high in refined carbohydrates and sugars can spike insulin levels, promoting fat storage. Conversely, diets rich in whole foods, lean proteins, and healthy fats support stable insulin levels and enhance fat burning.

Exercise: Regular physical activity, particularly a combination of cardiovascular exercise and strength training, is crucial for effective fat loss. Cardio burns calories during the activity, while strength training builds muscle, which increases your BMR.

Sleep and Stress: Adequate sleep and stress management are often overlooked but essential components of fat loss. Poor sleep and chronic stress can disrupt hormonal balance, increase appetite, and promote fat storage.

Practical Tips for Enhancing Fat Burning

To optimize fat burning and achieve your fat loss goals, consider these practical tips:

Create a Caloric Deficit: The most fundamental principle of fat loss is creating a caloric deficit, where you consume fewer calories than your body needs. This forces your body to use stored fat for energy. However, ensure the deficit isn't too extreme, as this can lead to muscle loss and other health issues.

Incorporate Strength Training: Building muscle through strength training increases your resting metabolic rate, meaning you burn more calories even at rest. Include compound exercises like squats, deadlifts, and bench presses for maximum muscle engagement.

Prioritize Protein: High-protein diets support muscle maintenance during fat loss, reduce appetite, and increase the thermic effect of food (the energy required to digest, absorb, and process nutrients). Aim for lean protein sources like chicken, fish, beans, and legumes.

Stay Active Throughout the Day: Beyond structured workouts, increase your daily activity levels. Simple actions like taking the stairs, walking instead of driving, and standing more often can boost your overall energy expenditure.

Practice Intermittent Fasting: Intermittent fasting involves cycling between periods of eating and fasting. This approach can help stabilize insulin levels, enhance fat burning, and simplify calorie control. Common methods include the 16/8 method (16 hours fasting, 8 hours eating) and the 5:2 method (eating normally for five days, significantly reducing calories for two non-consecutive days).

Real-World Example: Jane's Fat Loss Journey

Let's consider a real-world example to illustrate these principles. Jane, a 35-year-old office worker, decided to lose 20 pounds of excess body fat. Here's how she applied the knowledge of fat storage and burning:

Diet Adjustments: Jane replaced processed foods with whole foods, increasing her intake of vegetables, lean proteins, and healthy fats. She also reduced her portion sizes to create a moderate caloric deficit.

Exercise Routine: Jane incorporated a mix of cardio and strength training into her weekly routine. She started with three days of 30-minute cardio sessions (like brisk walking and cycling) and two days of full-body strength training.

Lifestyle Changes: Jane improved her sleep hygiene by establishing a regular bedtime and limiting screen time before bed. She also practiced stress-reducing activities like yoga and meditation.

Tracking Progress: Jane tracked her food intake and workouts using a fitness app. This helped her stay accountable and make necessary adjustments to her diet and exercise routine.

After three months of consistent effort, Jane successfully lost 15 pounds of body fat. She felt more energetic, confident, and healthier overall.

By understanding how the body stores and burns fat and applying practical strategies, you too can achieve your fat loss goals. In the next chapters, we'll explore more specific techniques and dietary approaches to optimize fat loss and enhance your overall fitness journey.

Role Of Metabolism In Fat Loss

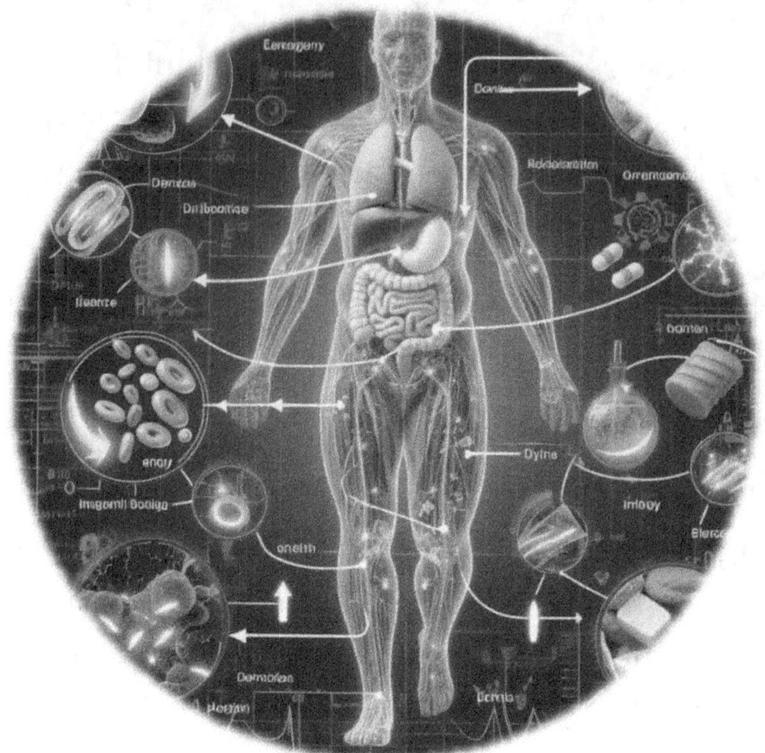

Metabolism is a complex process involving a series of chemical reactions within the body that convert food into energy. Understanding the role of metabolism in fat loss is crucial for creating an effective weight loss strategy. This chapter will explore how metabolism affects fat loss, the factors that influence metabolic rate, and practical ways to optimize your metabolism to achieve your fitness goals.

Understanding Metabolism

Metabolism is often thought of as a single process, but it actually comprises two main components: anabolism and catabolism.

Anabolism: This is the constructive phase of metabolism, where the body builds and stores compounds. For example, the synthesis of muscle proteins after a workout is an anabolic process.

Catabolism: This is the destructive phase of metabolism, where the body breaks down compounds to release energy. The breakdown of food during digestion and the subsequent release of energy for bodily functions are catabolic processes.

Together, these processes ensure that the body has a continuous supply of energy for growth, repair, and maintenance.

Basal Metabolic Rate (BMR)

The Basal Metabolic Rate (BMR) is the number of calories your body needs to perform basic physiological functions while at rest. These functions include breathing, circulating blood, and maintaining body temperature. BMR accounts for the majority of your daily caloric expenditure.

Several factors influence BMR:

Age: BMR decreases with age. As you get older, your body requires fewer calories to maintain basic functions.

Gender: Men generally have a higher BMR than women, primarily due to having more muscle mass.

Body Composition: Muscle tissue is more metabolically active than fat tissue. Therefore, individuals with higher muscle mass have a higher BMR.

Genetics: Genetic factors can influence metabolic rate, with some people naturally having a faster or slower metabolism.

Total Daily Energy Expenditure (TDEE)

Your Total Daily Energy Expenditure (TDEE) is the total number of calories you burn each day, including BMR and all physical activities. TDEE is influenced by three main components:

Basal Metabolic Rate (BMR): As mentioned, this is the energy required for basic bodily functions.

Thermic Effect of Food (TEF): This is the energy required to digest, absorb, and process the food you eat. TEF accounts for about 10% of your total caloric intake.

Physical Activity: This includes all movements, from walking and exercising to fidgeting. Physical activity can vary significantly between individuals, making it the most variable component of TDEE.

Metabolism and Fat Loss

To lose fat, you need to create a caloric deficit, where you consume fewer calories than your body needs, forcing it to use stored fat for energy. Understanding how metabolism works can help you create an effective fat loss strategy.

Caloric Deficit: Creating a caloric deficit is the foundation of fat loss. By consuming fewer calories than your TDEE, your body is forced to use stored fat for energy. However, it's essential to ensure that the deficit isn't too extreme, as this can lead to muscle loss and other health issues.

Muscle Preservation: Maintaining or building muscle mass is crucial during fat loss. Since muscle tissue is more metabolically active than fat tissue, having more muscle can increase your BMR, making it easier to sustain a caloric deficit. Strength training is an effective way to preserve muscle mass while losing fat.

Adaptive Thermogenesis: As you lose weight, your body can adapt by lowering its energy expenditure to conserve energy, a process known as adaptive thermogenesis. This can slow down your weight loss progress. To counter this, it's essential to adjust your caloric intake and exercise routine as you lose weight.

Factors Affecting Metabolic Rate

Several factors can influence your metabolic rate, either increasing or decreasing it. Understanding these factors can help you optimize your metabolism for fat loss.

Diet Composition: The macronutrient composition of your diet can affect your metabolic rate. Protein has a higher thermic effect than carbohydrates and fats, meaning your body burns more calories digesting and processing protein. Including more protein in your diet can help increase your metabolic rate.

Exercise: Physical activity is one of the most effective ways to boost your metabolism. Both aerobic (cardio) and anaerobic (strength training) exercises can increase your caloric expenditure. High-Intensity Interval Training (HIIT) is particularly effective at boosting metabolism due to the afterburn effect, where your body continues to burn calories even after the workout is over.

Hydration: Staying hydrated is essential for maintaining an optimal metabolic rate. Dehydration can slow down metabolism, making it harder to burn calories efficiently.

Sleep: Quality sleep is crucial for a healthy metabolism. Poor sleep can disrupt hormonal balance, leading to increased appetite and decreased energy expenditure. Aim for 7-9 hours of quality sleep per night to support your metabolic health.

Stress Management: Chronic stress can negatively impact metabolism by increasing the production of cortisol, a hormone that promotes fat storage, particularly around the abdomen. Incorporating stress-reducing activities like meditation, yoga, and deep breathing exercises can help maintain a healthy metabolism.

Practical Tips for Boosting Metabolism

Here are some practical tips to help you optimize your metabolism for fat loss:

Eat Protein-Rich Foods: Incorporate high-protein foods into your diet, such as lean meats, fish, eggs, dairy products, legumes, and nuts. Protein not only helps preserve muscle mass but also increases the thermic effect of food, boosting your metabolism.

Engage in Regular Exercise: Combine cardio and strength training exercises to maximize caloric expenditure. Aim for at least 150 minutes of moderate-intensity cardio or 75 minutes of high-intensity cardio per week, along with two to three strength training sessions.

Stay Hydrated: Drink plenty of water throughout the day to support metabolic processes. Aim for at least 8 cups (64 ounces) of water daily, and more if you're physically active.

Get Adequate Sleep: Prioritize sleep by establishing a regular sleep schedule and creating a relaxing bedtime routine. Aim for 7-9 hours of quality sleep per night.

Manage Stress: Incorporate stress-reducing activities into your daily routine. Techniques like deep breathing, meditation, and yoga can help lower cortisol levels and support a healthy metabolism.

Eat Small, Frequent Meals: Eating small, balanced meals throughout the day can help maintain steady energy levels and prevent overeating. Avoid skipping meals, as this can lead to overeating later in the day and negatively impact your metabolism.

Real-World Example: John's Metabolic Boost

Let's consider the example of John, a 40-year-old office worker who wanted to lose 30 pounds. Here's how he optimized his metabolism to achieve his fat loss goals:

Diet Adjustments: John increased his protein intake by including lean meats, fish, and legumes in his meals. He also reduced his consumption of processed foods and sugary beverages, focusing on whole, nutrient-dense foods.

Exercise Routine: John started with three days of moderate-intensity cardio (like brisk walking and cycling) and two days of strength training. As he progressed, he incorporated HIIT workouts to further boost his metabolism.

Hydration and Sleep: John made a conscious effort to drink more water throughout the day and improved his sleep hygiene by establishing a consistent bedtime routine.

Stress Management: To manage stress, John began practicing mindfulness meditation and yoga, which helped lower his cortisol levels and support his fat loss efforts.

Meal Frequency: John adopted a meal plan that included small, frequent meals to maintain steady energy levels and prevent overeating.

After six months of consistent effort, John successfully lost 25 pounds and significantly improved his overall health and well-being.

By understanding the role of metabolism in fat loss and implementing practical strategies to optimize it, you can achieve your weight loss goals more effectively. In the following chapters, we'll explore more advanced techniques and dietary approaches to further enhance your fat loss journey.

Impact Of Hormones On Fat Loss

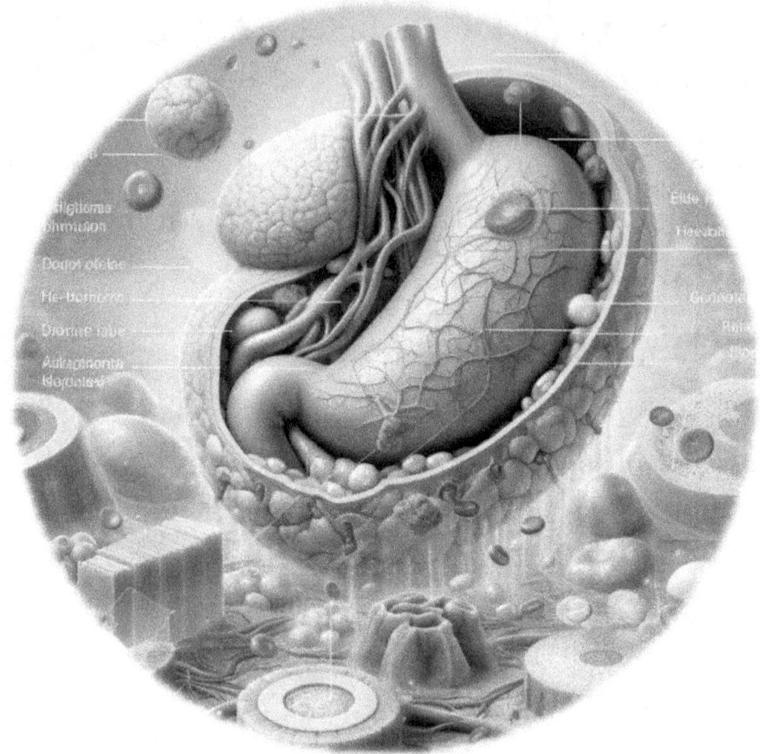

Hormones are the body's chemical messengers, playing a vital role in regulating numerous physiological processes, including fat loss. Understanding the impact of hormones on fat metabolism can provide valuable insights into effective weight management strategies. This chapter will explore the key hormones involved in fat loss, their functions, and practical ways to optimize hormonal balance to support your fat loss goals.

Key Hormones Involved in Fat Loss

Several hormones significantly influence fat storage and burning. Here are the primary hormones you need to understand:

Insulin:

Function: Insulin is produced by the pancreas and regulates blood sugar levels. It facilitates the uptake of glucose into cells for energy or storage as glycogen in the liver and muscles. Excess glucose is converted into fatty acids and stored as fat.

Impact on Fat Loss: High insulin levels promote fat storage and inhibit fat burning. Stable insulin levels are crucial for effective fat loss.

Glucagon:

Function: Also produced by the pancreas, glucagon works in opposition to insulin. It raises blood sugar levels by promoting the release of stored glucose from the liver.

Impact on Fat Loss: Glucagon stimulates the breakdown of glycogen and fat, making it an essential hormone for fat burning.

Leptin:

Function: Leptin is produced by fat cells and helps regulate energy balance by signaling the brain to reduce appetite and increase energy expenditure.

Impact on Fat Loss: High levels of leptin typically reduce hunger, but obesity can lead to leptin resistance, where the brain no longer responds effectively to leptin signals, hindering fat loss efforts.

Ghrelin:

Function: Known as the "hunger hormone," ghrelin is produced in the stomach and stimulates appetite.

Impact on Fat Loss: Elevated ghrelin levels increase hunger, making it challenging to maintain a caloric deficit necessary for fat loss.

Cortisol:

Function: Produced by the adrenal glands, cortisol is a stress hormone that helps the body respond to stress by increasing blood sugar levels and mobilizing energy.

Impact on Fat Loss: Chronic high levels of cortisol can lead to increased fat storage, particularly in the abdominal area, and muscle breakdown.

Thyroid Hormones (T3 and T4):

Function: The thyroid gland produces T3 (triiodothyronine) and T4 (thyroxine), which regulate metabolism.

Impact on Fat Loss: Optimal levels of thyroid hormones are essential for maintaining a healthy metabolic rate. Hypothyroidism (low thyroid function) can slow metabolism and make fat loss more difficult.

Practical Strategies to Optimize Hormonal Balance

Balancing these hormones can significantly enhance your fat loss efforts. Here are practical strategies to help you achieve hormonal balance:

Maintain Stable Blood Sugar Levels:

How: Eat balanced meals with a mix of protein, healthy fats, and complex carbohydrates. Avoid refined sugars and processed foods that cause rapid spikes in blood sugar and insulin levels.

Example: Instead of a sugary cereal for breakfast, opt for a bowl of oatmeal topped with nuts, seeds, and berries to keep your blood sugar stable.

Incorporate Protein-Rich Foods:

How: Protein helps regulate ghrelin and promotes the release of leptin, reducing hunger and increasing satiety.

Example: Include lean proteins like chicken, fish, tofu, and legumes in your meals.

Manage Stress:

How: Engage in stress-reducing activities like meditation, yoga, and deep breathing exercises to lower cortisol levels.

Example: Spend 10 minutes each morning meditating or practicing deep breathing to start your day with a sense of calm.

Get Adequate Sleep:

How: Aim for 7-9 hours of quality sleep per night to regulate leptin and ghrelin levels and support overall hormonal balance.

Example: Establish a consistent bedtime routine, such as turning off electronic devices an hour before bed and reading a book to unwind.

Exercise Regularly:

How: Engage in both aerobic (cardio) and anaerobic (strength training) exercises to boost metabolism and support hormonal balance.

Example: Combine 30 minutes of brisk walking with 20 minutes of strength training three times a week.

Support Thyroid Health:

How: Ensure adequate intake of nutrients essential for thyroid function, such as iodine, selenium, and zinc. Avoid excessive consumption of goitrogenic foods (like soy and cruciferous vegetables) if you have thyroid issues.

Example: Incorporate iodine-rich foods like seaweed and selenium-rich foods like Brazil nuts into your diet.

Real-World Example: Sarah's Hormonal Balance Journey

Consider Sarah, a 32-year-old marketing manager struggling with weight loss despite her efforts to eat healthily and exercise regularly. By understanding the impact of hormones on fat loss, she made the following adjustments:

Diet Adjustments: Sarah reduced her intake of refined sugars and processed foods, opting for balanced meals rich in protein, healthy fats, and complex carbohydrates. She noticed a significant improvement in her energy levels and reduced cravings.

Stress Management: Sarah started practicing yoga and mindfulness meditation daily. These practices helped lower her cortisol levels, resulting in better sleep and improved fat loss.

Sleep Hygiene: Sarah established a consistent bedtime routine, ensuring she got 8 hours of quality sleep each night. Improved sleep helped regulate her hunger hormones, reducing late-night snacking.

Regular Exercise: Sarah combined cardio and strength training exercises, working out five days a week. This balanced approach helped boost her metabolism and support hormonal balance.

Nutrient Intake: Sarah included iodine-rich seaweed snacks and selenium-rich Brazil nuts in her diet to support her thyroid health. She also took a multivitamin to ensure she was getting essential nutrients.

After six months, Sarah successfully lost 20 pounds and felt more energetic and balanced. By addressing hormonal imbalances, she was able to break through her weight loss plateau and achieve her goals.

Conclusion

Hormones play a pivotal role in regulating fat storage and burning. By understanding the impact of hormones on fat loss and implementing practical strategies to optimize hormonal balance, you can enhance your weight loss efforts and achieve lasting results. In the following chapters, we'll explore specific dietary and exercise approaches to further support your fat loss journey and help you build the perfect body.

Chapter 3: Nutrition Fundamentals

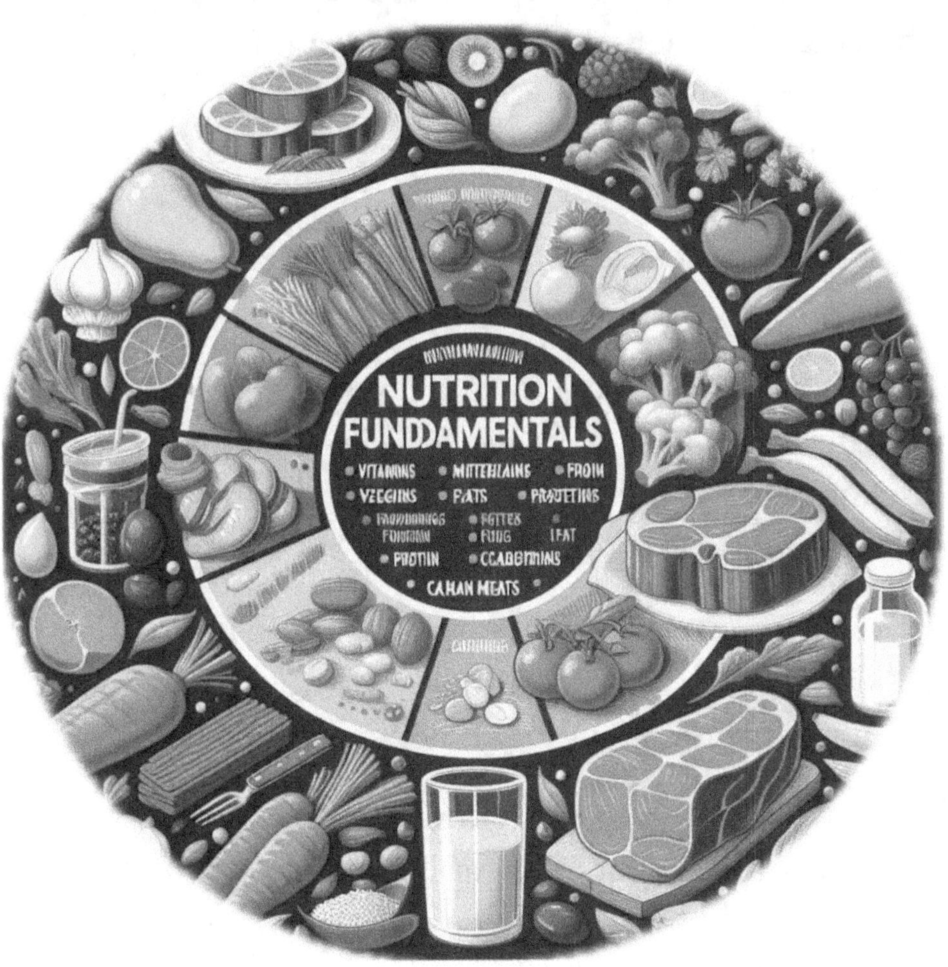

Macronutrients And Their Roles

Understanding macronutrients—carbohydrates, proteins, and fats—and their respective roles in the body is fundamental to designing an effective nutrition plan for achieving optimal body composition and performance. This chapter will delve into the functions of each macronutrient, their importance in supporting various bodily processes, and practical guidelines for incorporating them into your diet.

Carbohydrates: Fuel for Energy

Carbohydrates are the body's primary source of energy, particularly for high-intensity activities and brain function. They are classified into simple and complex carbohydrates based on their chemical structure.

Simple Carbohydrates: These are sugars that provide quick energy but lack nutritional value beyond calories. Examples include table sugar, honey, and fruit juices.

Complex Carbohydrates: Found in whole grains, vegetables, and legumes, complex carbs contain fiber, vitamins, and minerals. They provide sustained energy and support digestive health.

Role in the Body:

Energy Production: Carbohydrates are broken down into glucose, which fuels cellular processes and maintains blood sugar levels.

Brain Function: Glucose is crucial for cognitive function and concentration.

Muscle Glycogen: Carbohydrates are stored in muscles as glycogen, which is used during exercise to sustain endurance.

Example: Before a workout, consuming complex carbohydrates like oats or whole wheat toast can provide sustained energy for improved performance.

Proteins: Building Blocks of Tissue

Proteins are essential for building and repairing tissues, including muscles, organs, and the immune system. They are composed of amino acids, which are categorized into essential (obtained from food) and non-essential (produced by the body) amino acids.

Role in the Body:

Muscle Repair and Growth: Proteins are crucial for repairing and building muscle tissue, especially after exercise.

Enzyme Production: Enzymes, which facilitate biochemical reactions, are made from proteins.

Immune Function: Antibodies and immune cells rely on proteins to defend against infections.

Example: Consuming lean sources of protein such as chicken breast or tofu supports muscle recovery and maintenance.

Fats: Essential for Health

Fats are often misunderstood but are vital for overall health, providing energy, supporting cell growth, protecting organs, and maintaining body temperature. They are classified into saturated, unsaturated (monounsaturated and polyunsaturated), and trans fats.

Role in the Body:

Energy Storage: Fats provide a concentrated source of energy and are stored in adipose tissue.

Cell Membrane Structure: Fats are integral to cell membranes, influencing cellular function and signaling.

Hormone Production: Certain fats are used to produce hormones like testosterone and estrogen.

Example: Including sources of healthy fats such as avocados, nuts, and olive oil in your diet supports cardiovascular health and overall well-being.

Balancing Macronutrients for Optimal Nutrition

Achieving a balanced intake of macronutrients is essential for overall health and achieving fitness goals. Here are practical guidelines for balancing macronutrients in your diet:

Carbohydrates: Focus on whole grains, fruits, vegetables, and legumes for complex carbs. Limit intake of refined sugars and processed foods.

Proteins: Include lean meats, poultry, fish, eggs, dairy, legumes, and plant-based proteins like tofu and tempeh. Aim for a variety of sources to ensure adequate intake of essential amino acids.

Fats: Choose healthy fats such as avocados, nuts, seeds, olive oil, and fatty fish like salmon. Limit saturated and trans fats found in fried foods, baked goods, and processed snacks.

Practical Tips for Macronutrient Intake

Here are practical tips to help you optimize your macronutrient intake for health and performance:

Meal Planning: Plan meals that include a balance of all three macronutrients to support energy levels and satiety throughout the day.

Portion Control: Pay attention to portion sizes to avoid overconsumption of any macronutrient.

Timing: Adjust your macronutrient intake based on activity levels and goals. For example, consume more carbohydrates before exercise for energy or more protein after workouts for muscle repair.

Hydration: Drink adequate water throughout the day to support nutrient absorption and overall health.

Monitoring: Track your macronutrient intake using apps or food journals to ensure you're meeting your nutritional needs.

Real-World Example: Mark's Balanced Diet Approach

Consider Mark, a 28-year-old athlete aiming to improve his performance and body composition. Here's how he incorporates macronutrients into his diet:

Breakfast: Mark starts his day with oatmeal topped with berries and a scoop of protein powder for sustained energy and muscle repair.

Lunch: For lunch, Mark enjoys a grilled chicken salad with mixed greens, quinoa, and avocado for a balanced mix of protein, complex carbs, and healthy fats.

Snack: In the afternoon, Mark snacks on Greek yogurt with almonds and honey to boost protein intake and satisfy his hunger between meals.

Dinner: Dinner consists of baked salmon with steamed vegetables and a side of sweet potatoes for a nutrient-dense meal rich in protein, healthy fats, and complex carbs.

By understanding the roles of macronutrients and applying practical strategies to balance his diet, Mark supports his athletic performance and overall health goals effectively.

Conclusion

Macronutrients—carbohydrates, proteins, and fats—are essential for supporting various physiological functions and achieving optimal health and performance. By understanding their roles and incorporating them into a balanced diet, you can enhance your energy levels, support muscle growth and repair, and improve overall well-being. In the following chapters, we'll explore specific dietary strategies tailored to enhance muscle growth, reduce body fat, and optimize physical performance, helping you build the perfect body.

Importance Of Micronutrients

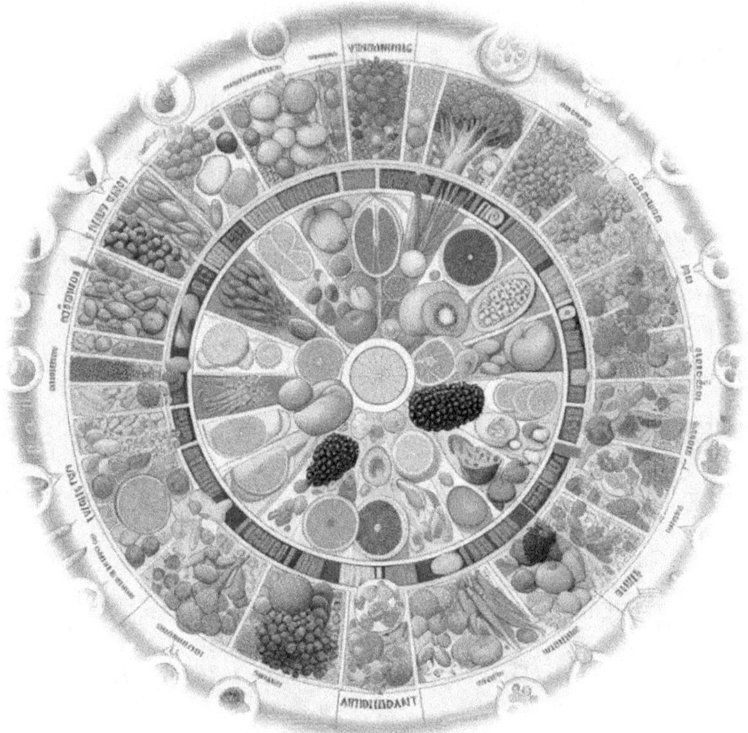

While macronutrients (carbohydrates, proteins, and fats) provide the body with energy and structural components, micronutrients play essential roles in supporting overall health, regulating metabolism, and maintaining cellular function. This chapter explores the significance of micronutrients, including vitamins and minerals, in optimizing health and enhancing physical performance.

Understanding Micronutrients

Micronutrients refer to vitamins and minerals that are required in small amounts but are critical for various physiological processes. They do not provide energy (calories) but are essential for energy metabolism, immune function, bone health, and countless biochemical reactions in the body.

Examples of Micronutrients:

Vitamins: Essential for growth, development, and overall health.

Vitamin C: Supports immune function and acts as an antioxidant (found in citrus fruits, strawberries, bell peppers).

Vitamin D: Critical for bone health and immune function (obtained from sunlight exposure and fortified foods like milk).

Vitamin B12: Necessary for nerve function and red blood cell production (found in animal products like meat, fish, and dairy).

Minerals: Important for bone health, fluid balance, nerve function, and muscle contraction.

Calcium: Essential for bone and teeth strength (found in dairy products, leafy greens, and fortified foods).

Iron: Needed for oxygen transport in the blood (found in lean meats, beans, and fortified cereals).

Magnesium: Supports muscle and nerve function, as well as energy production (found in nuts, seeds, and whole grains).

Roles of Micronutrients in the Body

Micronutrients play diverse roles in maintaining health and optimizing bodily functions:

Energy Metabolism: Many vitamins and minerals act as coenzymes or cofactors in metabolic pathways that convert food into energy.

Immune Function: Vitamins A, C, D, and E, as well as minerals like zinc and selenium, support immune system function and help protect against infections.

Bone Health: Calcium, vitamin D, vitamin K, and magnesium are crucial for maintaining strong bones and preventing osteoporosis.

Nerve Function: Minerals such as potassium, calcium, and magnesium play roles in nerve impulse transmission and muscle contraction.

Antioxidant Defense: Vitamins C and E, along with minerals like selenium and zinc, act as antioxidants that neutralize free radicals and protect cells from damage.

Consequences of Micronutrient Deficiencies

Deficiencies in micronutrients can lead to various health problems:

Vitamin D Deficiency: Increases the risk of bone disorders like osteoporosis and can impair immune function.

Iron Deficiency: Causes anemia, resulting in fatigue, weakness, and impaired cognitive function.

Vitamin B12 Deficiency: Leads to nerve damage, fatigue, and anemia.

Vitamin C Deficiency: Causes scurvy, characterized by fatigue, swollen gums, and skin hemorrhages.

Practical Tips for Micronutrient Intake

To ensure adequate micronutrient intake, consider the following tips:

Eat a Variety of Foods: Consume a diverse range of fruits, vegetables, whole grains, lean proteins, and dairy or dairy alternatives to obtain a broad spectrum of vitamins and minerals.

Focus on Colorful Foods: Brightly colored fruits and vegetables (e.g., berries, spinach, carrots) are rich in antioxidants and phytochemicals that support overall health.

Consider Supplementation: If you have specific dietary restrictions (e.g., vegetarian or vegan diets) or medical conditions that affect nutrient absorption, consult a healthcare provider about supplement options.

Cook Food Appropriately: Certain cooking methods can preserve or destroy micronutrients. Steam or lightly sauté vegetables to retain their vitamin and mineral content.

Real-World Example: Maria's Micronutrient-Rich Diet

Maria, a 35-year-old fitness enthusiast, focuses on maintaining a balanced diet rich in micronutrients:

Breakfast: Maria starts her day with a spinach and tomato omelet, providing vitamins A, C, and K, as well as minerals like iron and calcium.

Lunch: For lunch, Maria enjoys a quinoa salad with mixed greens, bell peppers, chickpeas, and avocado, offering a variety of vitamins (C, E) and minerals (magnesium, potassium)

Snack: In the afternoon, Maria snacks on Greek yogurt with berries and almonds, boosting her intake of calcium, vitamin D, and antioxidants.

Dinner: Maria's dinner includes grilled salmon with steamed broccoli and sweet potatoes, providing omega-3 fatty acids, vitamin D, and essential minerals like potassium and magnesium.

By incorporating nutrient-dense foods into her meals, Maria ensures she meets her micronutrient needs for optimal health and performance.

Conclusion

Micronutrients are essential for supporting overall health, regulating metabolism, and maintaining cellular function. By understanding the roles of vitamins and minerals and incorporating a variety of nutrient-dense foods into your diet, you can optimize your health, enhance physical performance, and prevent micronutrient deficiencies. In the following chapters, we'll explore specific dietary strategies and meal planning techniques to help you achieve your fitness goals and build the perfect body.

Calculating Your Caloric Needs

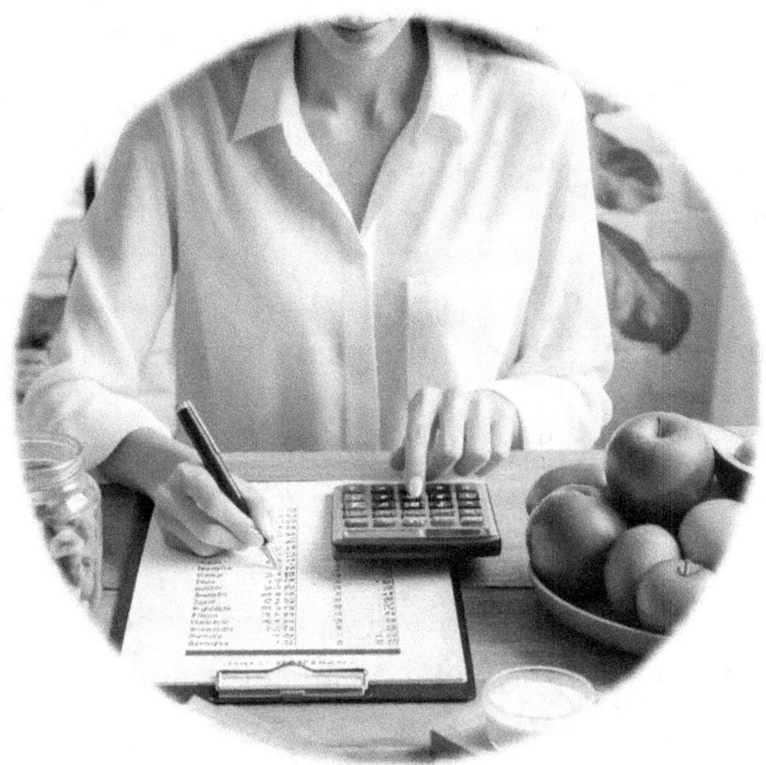

Understanding your caloric needs is essential for managing body weight, supporting physical activity, and achieving fitness goals. This chapter explores methods to calculate your daily caloric requirements, factors influencing calorie intake, and practical tips for maintaining a healthy balance.

Why Caloric Needs Matter

Calories are units of energy derived from food and beverages that the body uses to sustain vital functions and physical activity. Balancing calorie intake with expenditure is crucial for weight maintenance, loss, or gain, depending on individual goals.

Factors Influencing Caloric Needs:

Basal Metabolic Rate (BMR): The energy expended by the body at rest to maintain basic physiological functions like breathing and circulation.

Physical Activity Level: The amount of energy expended through exercise and daily activities.

Body Composition: Muscle mass requires more energy to maintain than fat tissue, influencing caloric needs.

Age and Gender: Metabolic rate tends to decrease with age, and men generally have higher calorie needs due to greater muscle mass.

Health Status: Certain medical conditions and medications can affect metabolism and energy requirements.

Methods to Calculate Caloric Needs

Several methods can estimate your daily caloric needs. Here are two commonly used approaches:

Harris-Benedict Equation:

For Men: BMR = 88.362 + (13.397 × weight in kg) + (4.799 × height in cm) - (5.677 × age in years)

For Women: BMR = 447.593 + (9.247 × weight in kg) + (3.098 × height in cm) - (4.330 × age in years)

Multiply BMR by an activity factor (ranging from sedentary to very active) to determine total daily energy expenditure (TDEE).

Mifflin-St Jeor Equation: An updated version of the Harris-Benedict equation that may be more accurate for some individuals.

Example Calculation:

Sarah is a 30-year-old female, 150 cm tall (5 feet), and weighs 60 kg (132 pounds).

Using the Harris-Benedict equation:

$$BMR = 447.593 + (9.247 \times 60) + (3.098 \times 150) - (4.330 \times 30)$$

$$BMR \approx 447.593 + 554.82 + 464.7 - 129.9$$

$$BMR \approx 1337.213 \text{ calories/day (rounded to 1337 calories/day)}$$

Adjusting Caloric Intake for Goals

Once you have estimated your daily caloric needs, you can adjust your intake based on your goals:

Weight Loss: Create a caloric deficit by consuming fewer calories than your TDEE, typically by 500-1000 calories/day for gradual, sustainable weight loss.

Weight Maintenance: Match your calorie intake to your TDEE.

Weight Gain: Consume more calories than your TDEE, focusing on nutrient-dense foods to support muscle growth.

Practical Tips for Caloric Management

Track Food Intake: Use apps or food journals to monitor your daily calorie intake and adjust as needed.

Focus on Nutrient Density: Choose whole, nutrient-dense foods like fruits, vegetables, lean proteins, and whole grains to meet your caloric needs while supporting overall health.

Consider Macronutrient Balance: Ensure your diet includes a balance of carbohydrates, proteins, and fats to optimize energy levels and support bodily functions.

Real-World Example: John's Caloric Management Strategy

John, a 40-year-old office worker looking to lose weight, follows these steps:

Calculate TDEE: Using the Mifflin-St Jeor equation, John estimates his TDEE at 2000 calories/day based on a sedentary lifestyle.

Create a Caloric Deficit: John aims to consume 1500 calories/day to create a deficit of 500 calories/day for steady weight loss.

Monitor Progress: John tracks his food intake using a calorie-tracking app and adjusts portions and food choices to stay within his calorie target.

Adjust as Needed: Depending on his progress, John adjusts his caloric intake and physical activity levels to achieve his weight loss goals effectively.

By understanding and managing his caloric needs, John maintains control over his weight management journey while ensuring he meets his nutritional requirements.

<u>Conclusion</u>

Calculating your caloric needs is a fundamental step in managing body weight, supporting physical activity, and achieving health and fitness goals. By estimating your daily energy requirements, adjusting your caloric intake based on your goals, and focusing on nutrient-dense foods, you can optimize your nutritional intake and promote overall well-being. In the following chapters, we'll explore specific dietary strategies and meal planning techniques to help you build the perfect body and maintain long-term health.

Chapter 4: The Importance Of Rest And Recovery

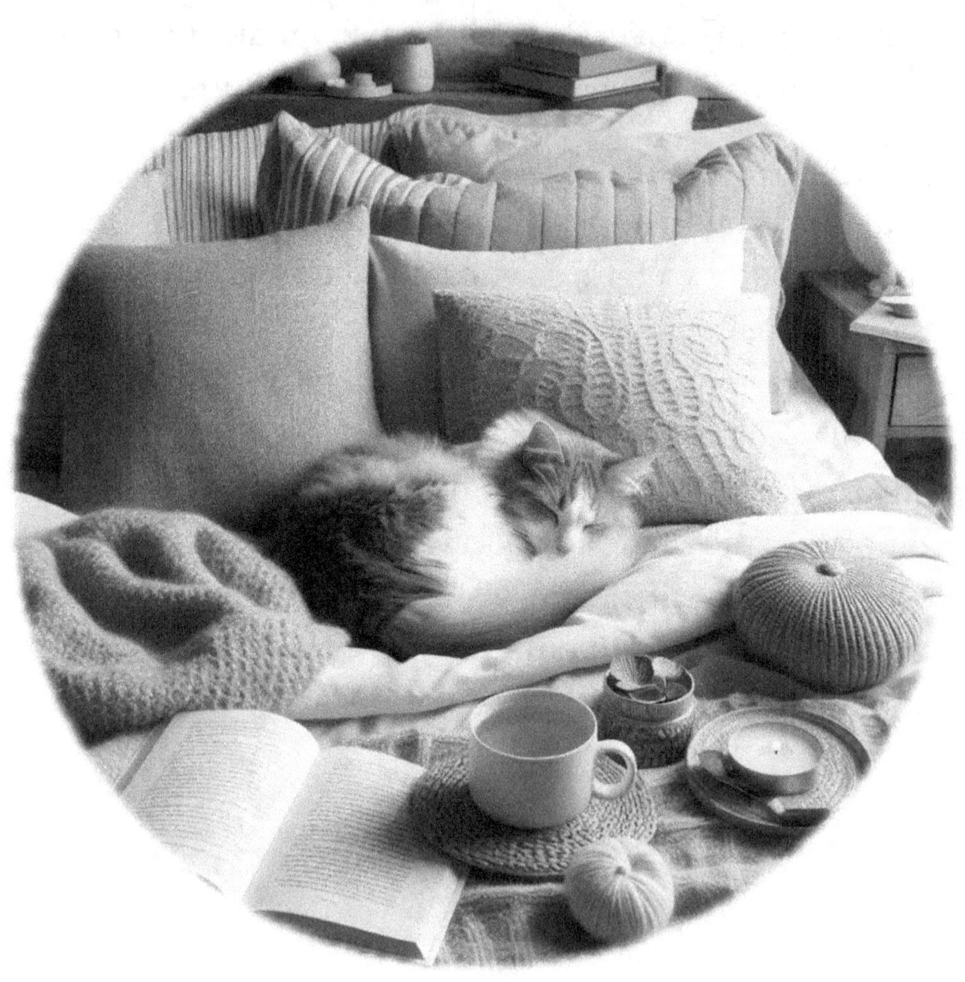

The Science Of Sleep And Muscle Recovery

Understanding the profound impact of sleep on muscle recovery is crucial for maximizing the benefits of your training efforts. This chapter explores the science behind sleep, its role in muscle repair and growth, and practical strategies to optimize your sleep for enhanced physical performance.

The Role of Sleep in Muscle Recovery

Sleep is a dynamic process essential for overall health and well-being, including the repair and growth of muscle tissue. During sleep, the body undergoes various physiological processes that are critical for recovery:

Hormone Regulation: Sleep supports the release of growth hormone, which plays a key role in tissue repair, muscle growth, and fat metabolism.

Muscle Repair: Adequate sleep allows for the repair of muscle fibers damaged during exercise, helping to enhance strength and endurance.

Energy Restoration: Sleep replenishes glycogen stores in muscles, providing energy for the next day's activities and workouts.

The Stages of Sleep

Sleep consists of several stages, each with distinct physiological functions:

Non-Rapid Eye Movement (NREM) Sleep:

Stage 1: Light sleep, transitioning between wakefulness and sleep.

Stage 2: Deeper sleep where heart rate and body temperature decrease.

Rapid Eye Movement (REM) Sleep: Associated with dreaming and essential for cognitive function and memory consolidation.

Example: A typical sleep cycle lasts about 90 minutes and includes multiple stages of NREM and REM sleep, repeating throughout the night.

Impact of Sleep Deprivation on Muscle Recovery

Insufficient sleep can impair muscle recovery and physical performance:

Reduced Growth Hormone Production: Inadequate sleep limits the release of growth hormone, hindering muscle repair and growth.

Increased Inflammation: Sleep deprivation can elevate markers of inflammation, delaying recovery and increasing injury risk.

Impaired Cognitive Function: Lack of sleep diminishes concentration, coordination, and decision-making abilities, impacting exercise performance.

Practical Strategies for Optimizing Sleep

To enhance muscle recovery and overall well-being, consider the following sleep optimization strategies:

Establish a Sleep Schedule: Maintain consistent sleep and wake times to regulate your body's internal clock.

Create a Sleep-Friendly Environment: Ensure your bedroom is cool, dark, and quiet to promote restful sleep.

Limit Screen Time: Reduce exposure to screens (phones, computers, TVs) before bedtime to promote melatonin production and improve sleep quality.

Practice Relaxation Techniques: Engage in relaxation practices such as deep breathing, meditation, or gentle stretching before bed to unwind and prepare for sleep.

Real-World Example: Sarah's Sleep Routine for Recovery

Sarah, a competitive athlete, prioritizes sleep to optimize her muscle recovery:

Consistent Bedtime: Sarah goes to bed and wakes up at the same time each day, maintaining a regular sleep schedule.

Sleep Environment: Her bedroom is equipped with blackout curtains, a comfortable mattress, and minimal noise to enhance sleep quality.

Pre-Bedtime Routine: Sarah practices relaxation techniques like yoga and deep breathing to relax her mind and body before sleep.

Sleep Tracking: She uses a sleep tracking app to monitor her sleep patterns and adjust her routine as needed for optimal recovery.

By prioritizing quality sleep, Sarah supports her muscle recovery, enhances her athletic performance, and maintains overall health.

Conclusion

Quality sleep is integral to muscle recovery, physical performance, and overall well-being. By understanding the science of sleep, implementing effective sleep strategies, and prioritizing restorative sleep habits, you can optimize muscle repair, support training adaptations, and achieve your fitness goals more effectively. In the following chapters, we'll explore additional strategies for enhancing recovery, nutrition tips for fueling your workouts, and practical guidance to help you build the perfect body.

Active Vs. Passive Recovery

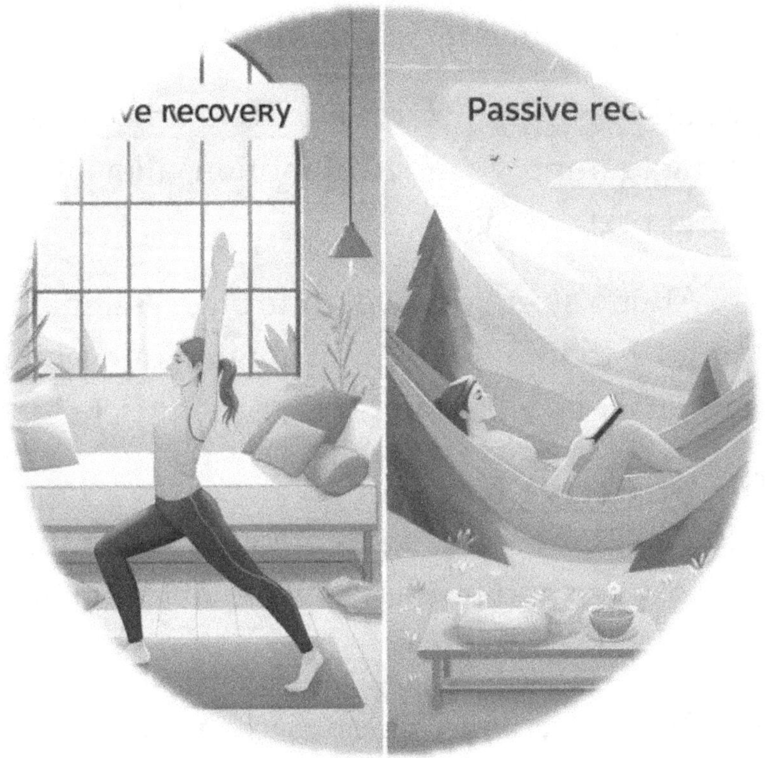

Rest and recovery are essential components of any effective training program, influencing your ability to perform optimally and achieve fitness goals. This chapter explores the concepts of active and passive recovery, their benefits, and how to integrate them into your fitness regimen for enhanced results.

Understanding Active Recovery

Active recovery involves engaging in low-intensity exercise or movement to promote circulation, reduce muscle stiffness, and enhance recovery without causing additional fatigue. Activities typically include:

Light Cardiovascular Exercise: Such as walking, cycling, or swimming at a comfortable pace to increase blood flow and promote nutrient delivery to muscles.

Mobility and Flexibility Exercises: Stretching, yoga, or foam rolling to improve range of motion, alleviate muscle tension, and prevent injury.

Example: After a strenuous weightlifting session, performing 10-15 minutes of light jogging or cycling helps flush out metabolic waste and facilitates muscle recovery.

Benefits of Active Recovery

Improved Circulation: Increases blood flow to muscles, delivering oxygen and nutrients essential for repair and growth.

Enhanced Muscle Repair: Promotes the removal of metabolic byproducts (e.g., lactic acid) that contribute to muscle soreness and fatigue.

Mental Refreshment: Light exercise can reduce stress levels and improve mood, aiding in overall recovery and readiness for subsequent workouts.

Understanding Passive Recovery

Passive recovery involves rest and minimal physical activity to allow the body to recuperate without additional stress. This approach typically includes:

Rest and Sleep: Allowing sufficient time for muscles to repair and regenerate during periods of sleep or rest days.

Hydration and Nutrition: Consuming adequate fluids and nutritious foods to support recovery processes, replenish glycogen stores, and repair muscle tissue.

Example: Taking a day off from intense training to rest, hydrate, and focus on nutrient-dense meals to support recovery from previous workouts.

Benefits of Passive Recovery

Muscle Regeneration: Allows for optimal repair of muscle tissue damaged during exercise, supporting strength and endurance gains over time.

Reduced Risk of Overtraining: Helps prevent burnout and reduces the risk of injury associated with excessive physical stress.

Energy Restoration: Allows the body to replenish energy stores (glycogen) and restore hormonal balance essential for recovery.

Integrating Both Approaches

To optimize recovery and performance, consider integrating both active and passive recovery strategies into your training regimen:

Balanced Approach: Alternate between days of moderate exercise and active recovery sessions (e.g., light cardio or mobility work).

Listen to Your Body: Pay attention to signs of fatigue, soreness, or decreased performance, adjusting your recovery strategy accordingly.

Periodization: Incorporate planned rest days or deload weeks into your training schedule to allow for comprehensive recovery and adaptation.

Real-World Example: James' Recovery Routine

James, a marathon runner, balances active and passive recovery to support his training:

Active Recovery: On days between long runs, James includes gentle stretching, yoga, and short walks to promote circulation and flexibility.

Passive Recovery: After intense training sessions or races, James prioritizes rest, adequate sleep, and hydration to allow his body to recover fully.

Nutrition Focus: James emphasizes nutrient-dense meals with a balance of carbohydrates, proteins, and fats to support muscle repair and replenish energy stores.

By incorporating both active and passive recovery strategies into his routine, James optimizes his recovery process, enhances performance, and reduces the risk of overuse injuries.

<u>Conclusion</u>

Active and passive recovery are integral components of an effective training program, influencing your ability to recover, adapt, and perform at your best. By understanding the benefits of each approach and integrating them into your fitness regimen, you can optimize muscle repair, prevent overtraining, and achieve your fitness goals more effectively. In the following chapters, we'll delve deeper into nutrition strategies, workout programming, and lifestyle factors to help you build the perfect body while prioritizing rest and recovery.

The Role Of Rest Days In Training Programs

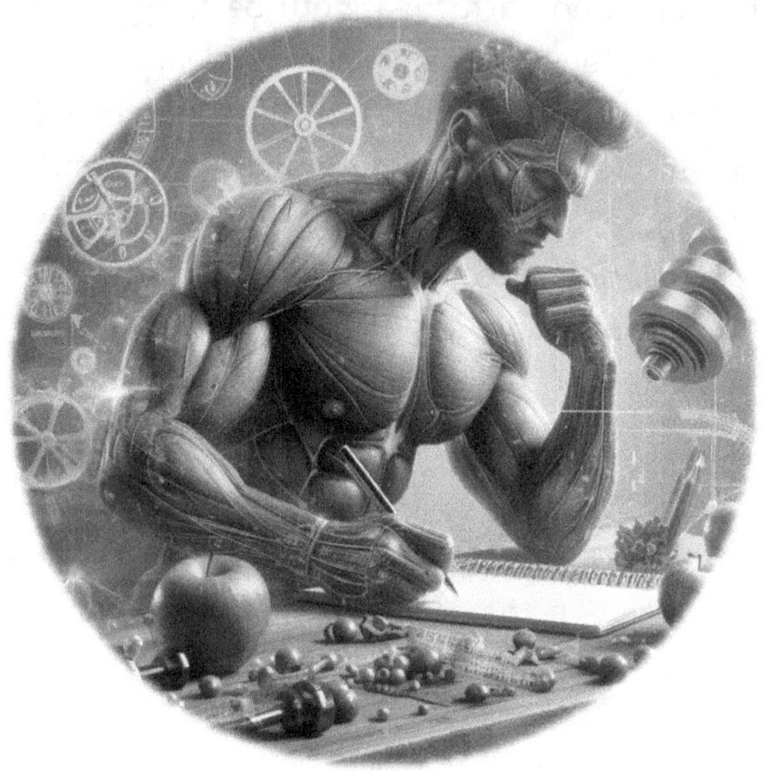

Rest days are crucial for optimizing performance, preventing injury, and achieving long-term fitness goals. This chapter explores the significance of rest days in training programs, their physiological benefits, and strategies for effective implementation to enhance overall fitness and well-being.

Understanding the Need for Rest Days

In the context of fitness and exercise, rest days refer to designated periods of reduced physical activity or complete rest. These periods allow the body to recover from intense workouts, adapt to training stimuli, and rebuild stronger muscle tissue.

Example: After a week of intense weightlifting sessions targeting various muscle groups, taking a rest day allows muscles time to repair and grow, optimizing strength gains.

Physiological Benefits of Rest Days

Rest days provide several physiological benefits essential for maximizing training adaptations and overall performance:

Muscle Repair and Growth: During rest, muscles repair microscopic tears and increase in size (hypertrophy) in response to resistance training stimuli.

Energy Restoration: Allows replenishment of glycogen stores in muscles and liver, essential for sustained energy during workouts.

Central Nervous System Recovery: Reduces mental and physical fatigue, enhancing coordination, reaction times, and overall performance.

Preventing Overtraining and Injury

Overtraining occurs when the body is subjected to excessive exercise without adequate recovery, leading to fatigue, decreased performance, and increased injury risk. Rest days help mitigate these risks by:

Preventing Burnout: Allows mental and physical rejuvenation, reducing the likelihood of burnout and maintaining motivation.

Reducing Injury Risk: Provides time for tissues (muscles, tendons, ligaments) to repair and strengthen, minimizing the risk of overuse injuries.

Optimizing Training Adaptations

Integrating regular rest days into your training program optimizes the body's ability to adapt to exercise stimuli, leading to:

Improved Performance: Enhances strength, endurance, and speed as muscles recover and rebuild stronger.

Consistent Progress: Facilitates long-term progress by balancing workout intensity with adequate recovery periods.

Strategies for Effective Rest Day Implementation

To maximize the benefits of rest days in your training program, consider the following strategies:

Scheduled Rest Days: Plan specific days each week dedicated to rest or active recovery (e.g., light stretching, yoga, or leisurely activities).

Listen to Your Body: Pay attention to signs of fatigue, soreness, or decreased performance, adjusting your rest day frequency or intensity as needed.

Active Recovery: Incorporate low-intensity activities like walking, swimming, or gentle stretching on rest days to promote circulation and flexibility.

Real-World Example: Emily's Training Schedule

Emily, a competitive cyclist, structures her training week to include strategic rest days:

Intensity Variation: Alternates between high-intensity cycling sessions and rest days to allow her muscles to recover and adapt.

Active Recovery: On rest days, Emily enjoys leisurely walks or engages in yoga to maintain flexibility and promote recovery.

Nutrition Focus: Emily emphasizes nutrient-dense meals with adequate protein and carbohydrates to support muscle repair and energy replenishment on rest days.

By incorporating planned rest days into her training regimen, Emily enhances her cycling performance, reduces the risk of overtraining, and maintains overall health.

Conclusion

Rest days play a vital role in optimizing performance, preventing overtraining, and supporting long-term fitness goals. By understanding the physiological benefits of rest days and implementing effective strategies for their integration into your training program, you can enhance muscle recovery, improve training adaptations, and achieve sustainable progress. In the following chapters, we'll explore additional factors such as nutrition, recovery techniques, and workout programming to help you build the perfect body while prioritizing rest and recovery.

Chapter 5: Setting Realistic Goals

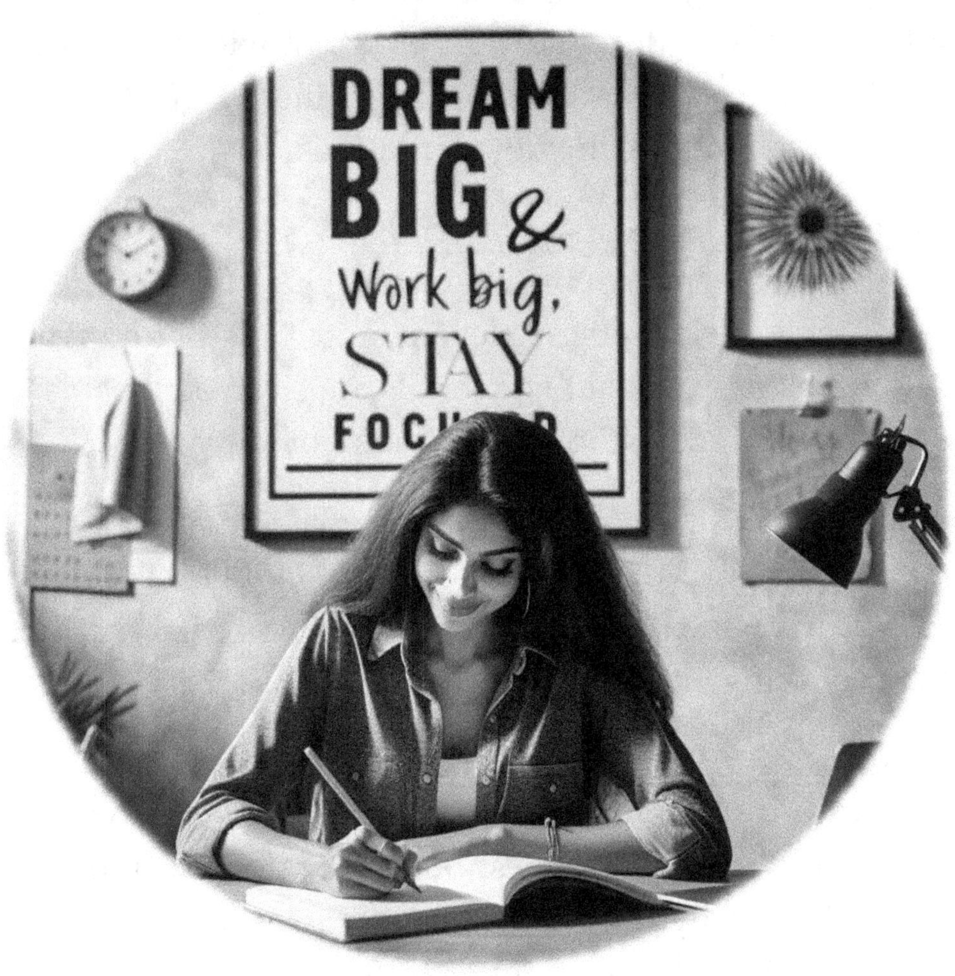

SMART Goals For Fitness

Setting effective goals is essential for guiding your fitness journey, maintaining motivation, and achieving sustainable progress. This chapter explores the concept of SMART goals in the context of fitness, providing practical insights and examples to help you set meaningful objectives aligned with your aspirations.

Understanding SMART Goals

SMART is an acronym that stands for Specific, Measurable, Achievable, Relevant, and Time-bound. This framework ensures that your goals are clear, actionable, and realistic, increasing the likelihood of success.

Example: Instead of setting a vague goal like "I want to lose weight," a SMART goal would be "I will lose 10 pounds in the next 3 months by following a balanced diet and exercising 4 times per week."

Components of SMART Goals

Specific: Clearly define what you want to achieve. Your goal should answer the questions: What do I want to accomplish? Why is this goal important? Who is involved? Where will it happen? What are the requirements and constraints?

Example: "I want to increase my bench press by 20 pounds within the next 8 weeks."

Measurable: Establish criteria for tracking progress and determining when you have achieved your goal. Include specific metrics or milestones that can be objectively measured.

Example: "I will track my progress by recording my bench press weight each week to ensure I am on track to increase by 20 pounds."

Achievable: Set goals that are challenging yet realistic given your current capabilities, resources, and time constraints. Ensure they stretch your abilities but are still within reach with effort and commitment.

Example: "I will increase my bench press gradually by 2.5 pounds per week, focusing on proper form and technique to avoid injury."

Relevant: Align your goals with your overall objectives and priorities. They should be meaningful and directly contribute to your long-term vision for health, fitness, or performance improvement.

Example: "Improving my bench press strength aligns with my goal of enhancing upper body muscular endurance and overall strength for my fitness competitions."

Time-bound: Set a deadline or timeframe for achieving your goal. This creates a sense of urgency and helps you stay focused and motivated.

Example: "I will achieve my goal of increasing my bench press by 20 pounds within the next 8 weeks, starting from today."

Benefits of SMART Goals in Fitness

Clarity and Focus: Clearly defined goals provide a roadmap for your fitness journey, reducing ambiguity and increasing motivation.

Progress Tracking: Measurable criteria allow you to track your progress systematically, celebrate achievements, and adjust strategies as needed.

Motivation and Commitment: Setting achievable yet challenging goals enhances commitment and persistence, driving continuous improvement.

Real-World Example: Jake's SMART Goal Journey

Jake, an aspiring marathon runner, sets a SMART goal to improve his race time:

Specific: "I will complete my next marathon in under 4 hours."

Measurable: "I will track my training runs and race times to monitor progress."

Achievable: "I will follow a structured training plan and gradually increase mileage to build endurance."

Relevant: "Improving my marathon time aligns with my goal of qualifying for a prestigious race next year."

Time-bound: "I will achieve this goal within the next 6 months, starting from today."

By adhering to the SMART criteria, Jake focuses his efforts, stays motivated throughout his training, and ultimately achieves his goal of running a marathon under 4 hours.

Conclusion

SMART goals provide a powerful framework for setting and achieving meaningful objectives in your fitness journey. By applying the principles of Specificity, Measurability, Achievability, Relevance, and Time-bound planning, you can clarify your aspirations, track progress effectively, and maintain motivation for long-term success. In the following chapters, we'll delve deeper into strategies for overcoming challenges, maintaining consistency, and fine-tuning your approach to build the perfect body and achieve your fitness aspirations.

Tracking Progress And Making Adjustments

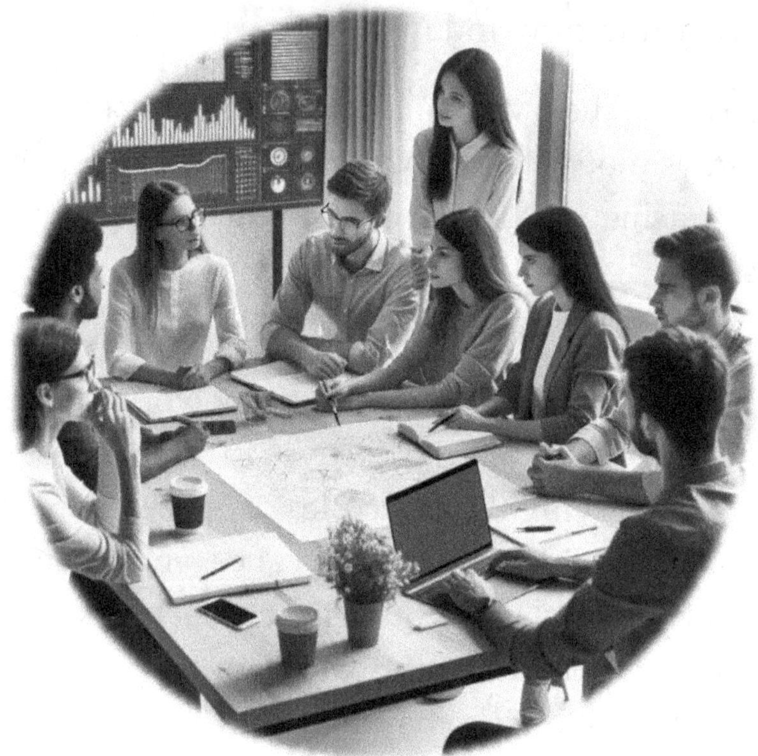

Tracking your progress and making adjustments are integral to achieving your fitness goals effectively and sustainably. This chapter explores practical strategies for monitoring progress, evaluating outcomes, and adapting your approach to ensure continued success on your fitness journey.

Importance of Tracking Progress

Tracking progress provides valuable insights into your journey towards achieving fitness goals:

Visibility: Allows you to see where you started, where you are, and how far you've come, providing motivation and a sense of accomplishment.

Accountability: Keeps you accountable to yourself, ensuring you stay committed to your goals and maintain consistency in your efforts.

Identification of Trends: Helps identify patterns in your behavior, training, and nutrition that impact your progress positively or negatively.

Methods for Tracking Progress

Measurement Metrics: Use quantifiable measures such as weight, body measurements (waist, hips, etc.), body fat percentage, or performance metrics (e.g., lifting weights, running times) to track changes over time.

Fitness Apps and Devices: Utilize fitness tracking apps or wearable devices that monitor activities, calories burned, sleep patterns, and other relevant metrics to provide real-time feedback.

Training Logs: Maintain a training journal or log to record workouts, sets, repetitions, and notes on how you felt during each session, allowing for reflection and adjustment.

Example: Tracking Weight Loss Progress

Sarah sets a goal to lose 20 pounds in 6 months. She tracks her progress using a combination of weekly weigh-ins and body measurements. After 3 months, Sarah has lost 12 pounds and notices a decrease in her waist measurement by 2 inches. This positive trend motivates her to continue following her nutrition plan and workout routine.

Evaluating Outcomes

Regularly evaluate your progress against your initial goals and timelines:

Assess Achievements: Celebrate milestones and achievements reached along the way to maintain motivation and reinforce positive behaviors.

Identify Challenges: Recognize barriers or challenges that may have hindered progress, such as inconsistent workouts, unhealthy eating habits, or external factors.

Adjust Goals as Needed: If progress is slower than expected or circumstances change, be flexible in adjusting your goals and timelines to remain realistic and achievable.

Making Adjustments

Based on your progress evaluation, make necessary adjustments to your approach:

Nutrition: Modify your diet to better support your goals, such as adjusting calorie intake, macronutrient ratios, or meal timing.

Training: Adjust workout intensity, frequency, or exercises to address weaknesses, plateaus, or changing fitness levels.

Rest and Recovery: Increase focus on recovery strategies, such as incorporating more rest days, improving sleep quality, or trying different recovery techniques (e.g., foam rolling, stretching).

Real-World Example: John's Progress Tracking and Adjustment

John aims to increase his squat strength by 50 pounds in 3 months. After the first month, he tracks his progress through strength gains recorded in his training log. Despite consistent effort, John notices his progress has plateaued. To overcome this, he adjusts his training program by incorporating more lower body accessory exercises and increasing his protein intake to support muscle recovery and growth. These adjustments lead to renewed progress towards his strength goal.

Conclusion

Tracking progress and making adjustments are essential practices in achieving and maintaining fitness goals. By regularly monitoring your progress, evaluating outcomes, and adapting your approach based on insights gained, you can optimize your efforts, overcome challenges, and sustain long-term success on your fitness journey. In the following chapters, we'll explore additional strategies for overcoming obstacles, maintaining motivation, and refining your approach to building the perfect body and achieving your fitness aspirations.

The Psychology Of Goal Setting

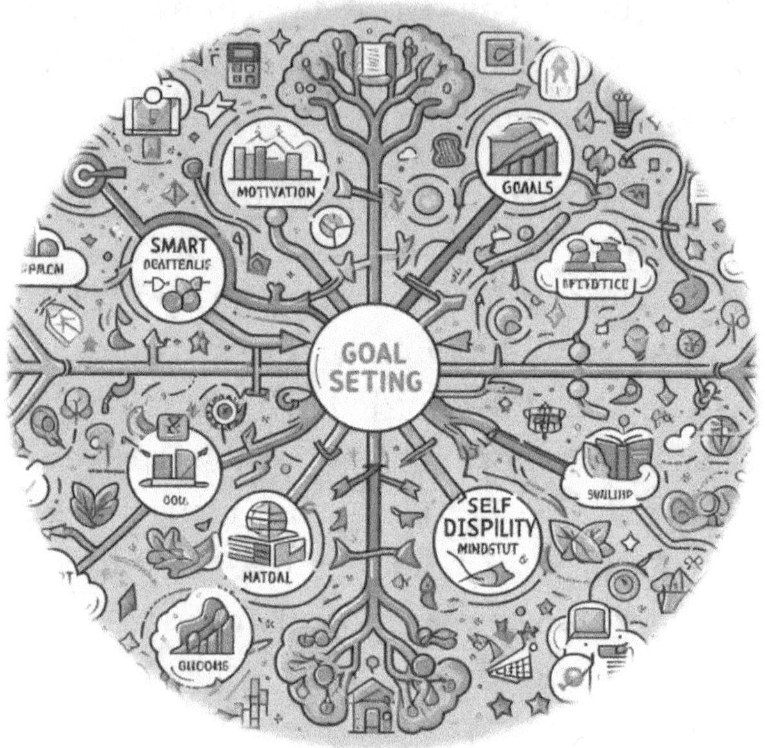

Understanding the psychology behind goal setting is crucial for effectively shaping behaviors, maintaining motivation, and achieving sustainable progress on your fitness journey. This chapter explores key psychological principles and strategies to help you set meaningful and achievable goals.

Motivation and Goal Setting

Motivation serves as the driving force behind goal setting and attainment:

Intrinsic vs. Extrinsic Motivation: Intrinsic motivation arises from internal desires and personal satisfaction (e.g., enjoyment of exercise), while extrinsic motivation comes from external rewards (e.g., praise, recognition).

Goal Orientation: People with a mastery orientation focus on improving skills and mastering tasks, while those with a performance orientation aim to outperform others or demonstrate competence.

Example: Sarah's Intrinsic Motivation

Sarah is intrinsically motivated to improve her fitness because she enjoys the challenge of strength training and the sense of accomplishment after completing tough workouts. This internal drive keeps her consistently engaged in her fitness goals.

Setting Effective Goals

Effective goal setting involves applying the SMART criteria (Specific, Measurable, Achievable, Relevant, Time-bound) to create clear objectives:

Specific: Define precisely what you want to achieve and why it matters to you. Clear goals provide direction and focus.

Measurable: Establish criteria for tracking progress and determining success. Measurable goals allow you to monitor your advancement.

Achievable: Set realistic goals that stretch your abilities but remain within reach with effort and commitment.

Relevant: Ensure your goals align with your values, aspirations, and long-term objectives. Relevant goals maintain relevance and meaning.

Time-bound: Set deadlines or timeframes for achieving your goals. This creates a sense of urgency and helps you prioritize tasks.

Example: John's SMART Goal

John sets a SMART goal to run a half-marathon in 6 months. His goal is specific (complete a half-marathon), measurable (by finishing the race), achievable (based on his current fitness level), relevant (supports his desire to improve cardiovascular health), and time-bound (within 6 months).

The Role of Self-Efficacy

Self-efficacy, or belief in one's ability to succeed, influences goal setting and achievement:

Building Confidence: Setting and achieving small, incremental goals can enhance self-efficacy and build confidence in your ability to tackle larger challenges.

Overcoming Setbacks: High self-efficacy helps individuals persist in the face of setbacks, viewing failures as learning opportunities rather than reasons to give up.

Example: Building Self-Efficacy

By progressively increasing the weight lifted during strength training sessions, Jake builds confidence in his ability to handle heavier loads and achieve his strength goals over time.

Goal Commitment and Persistence

Commitment to goals and persistence through challenges are crucial for long-term success:

Goal Commitment: Establishing a strong commitment to your goals increases motivation and dedication to achieving them.

Resilience: Resilience enables individuals to bounce back from setbacks, adapt to changes, and stay focused on their goals despite obstacles.

Example: Staying Committed

Emily faces a setback when she misses a week of training due to illness. Despite this, she maintains her commitment by adjusting her schedule and gradually easing back into her workouts, demonstrating resilience in pursuing her fitness goals.

Conclusion

The psychology of goal setting encompasses motivation, effective goal setting techniques, self-efficacy, and resilience—all essential components in achieving and sustaining progress on your fitness journey. By understanding these psychological principles and applying them to your goal-setting process, you can enhance motivation, overcome challenges, and achieve meaningful results. In the following chapters, we'll explore practical strategies for maintaining momentum, refining your approach, and achieving the perfect body while staying mentally resilient and focused on your goals.

Part 2: Building Muscle Mass

Chapter 6: Designing an Effective Workout Program

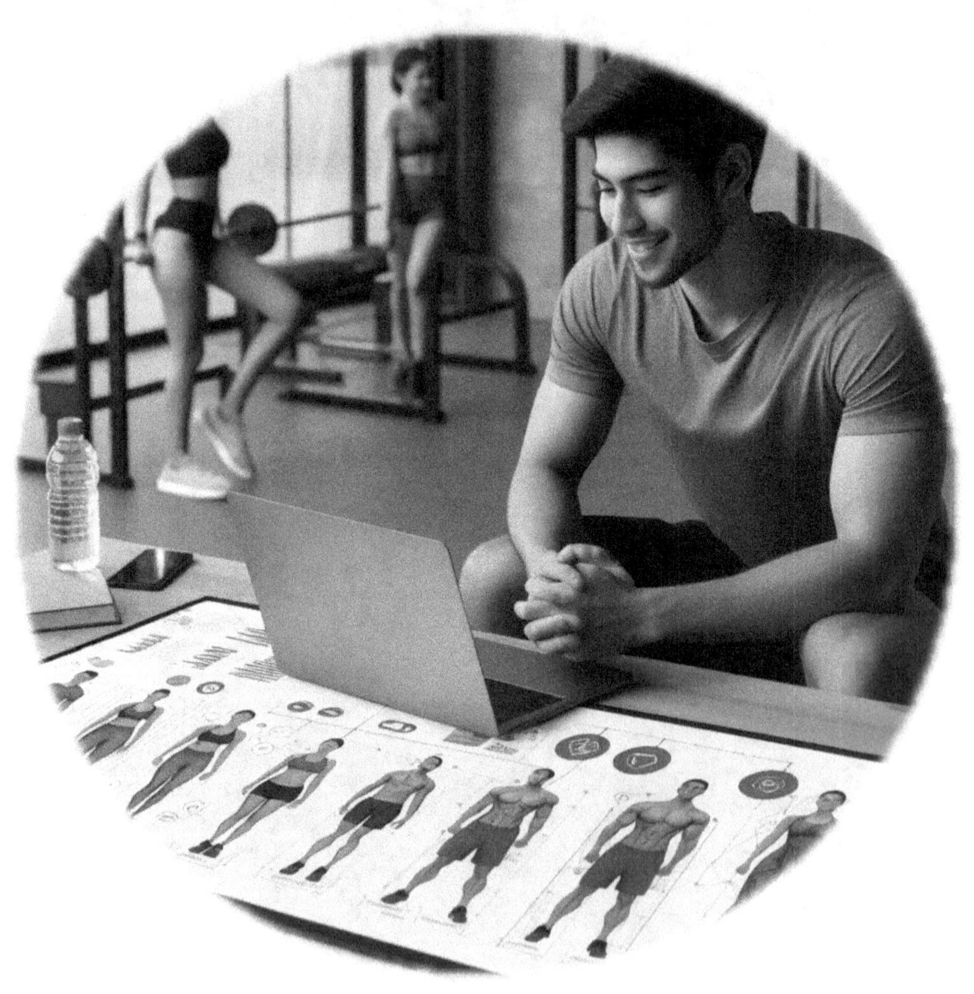

Key Components Of A Muscle-Building Program

Designing an effective muscle-building program requires careful consideration of various components to maximize hypertrophy, strength gains, and overall fitness. This chapter explores essential elements and strategies for creating a structured workout program focused on building lean muscle mass.

Understanding Muscle Hypertrophy

Muscle hypertrophy refers to the increase in muscle size and cross-sectional area, achieved primarily through resistance training and proper nutrition. Key principles include:

Progressive Overload: Gradually increasing the intensity, volume, or resistance of exercises to continually challenge muscles and stimulate growth.

Muscle Damage and Repair: Microscopic tears in muscle fibers during exercise trigger repair and growth processes, leading to hypertrophy.

Example: Progressive Overload

Sarah incorporates progressive overload into her strength training program by gradually increasing the weight lifted during squats each week, stimulating muscle adaptation and growth.

Components of a Muscle-Building Program

Resistance Training: Focus on compound exercises (e.g., squats, deadlifts, bench press) that target major muscle groups to promote overall strength and hypertrophy.

Example: A full-body workout routine includes exercises like barbell squats, pull-ups, and shoulder presses to engage multiple muscle groups effectively.

Volume and Intensity: Structuring workouts to include sufficient volume (sets and repetitions) and intensity (weight lifted) to induce muscle fatigue and stimulate growth.

Example: Performing 3-4 sets of 8-12 repetitions per exercise at 70-85% of your one-repetition maximum (1RM) for optimal hypertrophy.

Progression Strategies: Implementing techniques such as increasing weight, adjusting rest intervals, or varying exercise selection to ensure ongoing muscle adaptation.

Example: Periodically increasing the weight lifted during bicep curls or reducing rest periods between sets to enhance workout intensity and progression.

Rest and Recovery: Allowing adequate rest between workouts and prioritizing sleep and nutrition to support muscle repair and growth.

Example: Taking 48-72 hours of recovery between training sessions targeting the same muscle groups to optimize recovery and minimize injury risk.

Nutrition and Hydration: Consuming a balanced diet rich in protein, carbohydrates, and healthy fats to support muscle repair, energy levels, and overall performance.

Example: Including lean proteins (e.g., chicken breast, tofu), complex carbohydrates (e.g., quinoa, sweet potatoes), and sufficient water intake to fuel workouts and aid recovery.

Example Workout Program: Upper-Lower Split

Day 1: Upper Body

Bench Press: 4 sets x 8-10 reps

Pull-Ups: 3 sets x max reps

Overhead Press: 3 sets x 8-10 reps

Bent-Over Rows: 4 sets x 8-12 reps

Bicep Curls: 3 sets x 10-12 reps

Tricep Dips: 3 sets x 10-12 reps

Day 2: Lower Body

Squats: 4 sets x 8-10 reps

Deadlifts: 3 sets x 6-8 reps

Lunges: 3 sets x 12 reps each leg

Leg Press: 3 sets x 10-12 reps

Calf Raises: 4 sets x 15 reps

Integrating Periodization

Periodization involves varying workout parameters (volume, intensity, exercise selection) over time to prevent plateaus and promote continual progress:

Example: Cycling through phases of hypertrophy (high volume, moderate intensity), strength (moderate volume, high intensity), and recovery (deload weeks) to optimize muscle adaptation and performance.

Conclusion

Designing an effective muscle-building program involves integrating resistance training, volume and intensity management, progression strategies, adequate rest and recovery, and proper nutrition. By structuring your workouts around these key components and implementing progressive overload and periodization techniques, you can optimize muscle growth, strength gains, and overall fitness. In the following chapters, we'll explore advanced training techniques, recovery strategies, and nutritional considerations to further enhance your muscle-building journey and achieve the perfect body.

Split Routines Vs. Full-Body Workouts

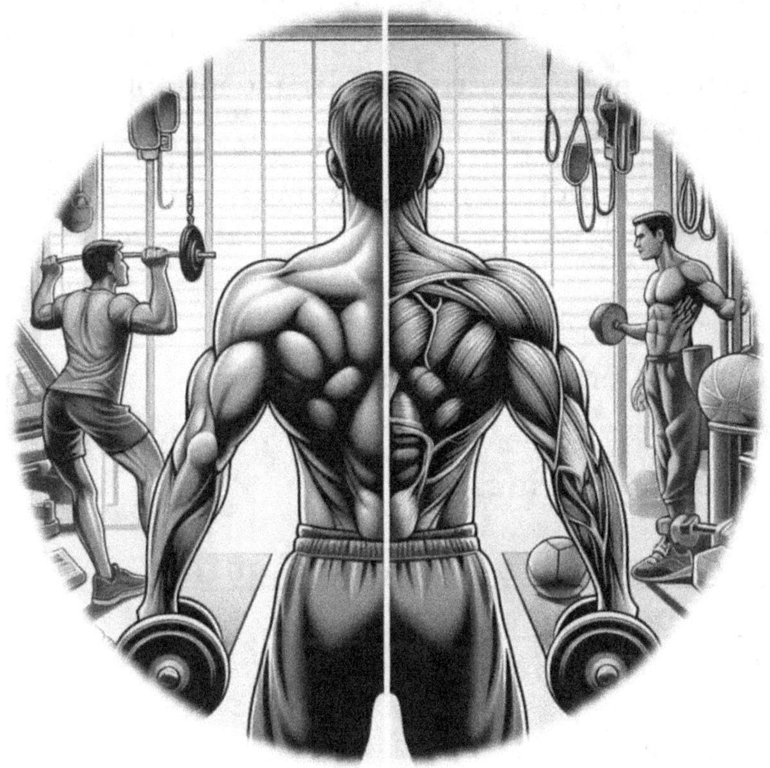

When designing a workout program, one of the key decisions you'll face is whether to follow a split routine or opt for full-body workouts. Each approach has its advantages and is suited to different fitness goals and schedules. This chapter explores the differences between split routines and full-body workouts, helping you determine which approach aligns best with your fitness objectives.

Understanding Split Routines

Split routines involve dividing your workouts to target specific muscle groups on different days of the week. Common split routines include:

Upper-Lower Split: Alternating between workouts that focus on upper body muscles (chest, back, shoulders, arms) and lower body muscles (quadriceps, hamstrings, calves).

Push-Pull-Legs Split: Grouping exercises based on movement patterns — push exercises (chest, shoulders, triceps), pull exercises (back, biceps), and leg exercises (quadriceps, hamstrings, calves).

Example: Upper-Lower Split Routine
Day 1: Upper Body
Bench Press (4 sets x 8-10 reps)

Pull-Ups (3 sets x max reps)

Overhead Press (3 sets x 8-10 reps)

Bent-Over Rows (4 sets x 8-12 reps)

Bicep Curls (3 sets x 10-12 reps)

Tricep Dips (3 sets x 10-12 reps)

Day 2: Lower Body
Squats (4 sets x 8-10 reps)

Deadlifts (3 sets x 6-8 reps)

Lunges (3 sets x 12 reps each leg)

Leg Press (3 sets x 10-12 reps)

Calf Raises (4 sets x 15 reps)

Benefits of Split Routines

Targeted Muscle Focus: Allows you to concentrate on specific muscle groups during each workout, optimizing muscle stimulation and growth.

Recovery: Provides adequate recovery time for muscles between sessions targeting the same muscle group, reducing the risk of overtraining.

Flexibility: Offers flexibility in workout structure and allows customization based on individual goals and preferences.

Understanding Full-Body Workouts

Full-body workouts involve training all major muscle groups in a single session. This approach typically includes compound exercises that engage multiple muscles simultaneously.

Example: Full-Body Workout

Squats (3 sets x 10 reps)

Bench Press (3 sets x 10 reps)

Pull-Ups (3 sets x max reps)

Deadlifts (3 sets x 8 reps)

Overhead Press (3 sets x 10 reps)

Plank (3 sets x 30 seconds)

Benefits of Full-Body Workouts

Efficiency: Maximizes time efficiency by targeting all major muscle groups in one session, ideal for individuals with limited time for workouts.

Frequency: Allows for more frequent training of each muscle group throughout the week, promoting muscle development and metabolic benefits.

Overall Fitness: Enhances overall strength, endurance, and functional fitness by integrating multiple movement patterns in each workout.

Choosing the Best Approach

When deciding between split routines and full-body workouts, consider the following factors:

Fitness Goals: If your goal is to specialize in specific muscle groups or improve strength in particular areas, a split routine may be more appropriate.

Time Availability: Full-body workouts are beneficial for individuals with busy schedules, as they require fewer sessions per week to train all muscle groups.

Recovery Needs: Assess your recovery capacity and prioritize adequate rest between workouts, especially if following a split routine targeting the same muscle groups frequently.

Real-World Example: Sarah's Training Approach

Sarah prefers a full-body workout routine three times a week due to her hectic work schedule. This allows her to maintain overall fitness and strength while accommodating her busy lifestyle.

Conclusion

Both split routines and full-body workouts can be effective approaches to designing a workout program, depending on your goals, preferences, and schedule. By understanding the differences, benefits, and considerations of each approach, you can tailor your training regimen to optimize muscle growth, strength gains, and overall fitness. In the following chapters, we'll delve deeper into advanced training techniques, recovery strategies, and nutritional considerations to further enhance your workout program and help you achieve the perfect body.

Periodization Techniques

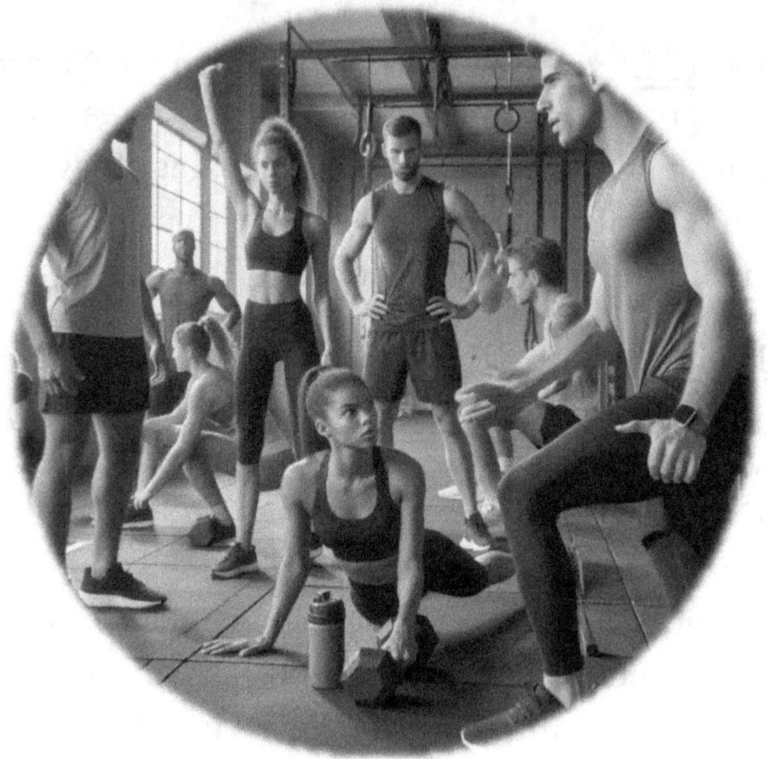

Periodization is a strategic approach to training that involves varying workout variables over time to maximize performance, prevent plateaus, and reduce the risk of overtraining. This chapter explores different periodization techniques and how you can integrate them into your workout program to achieve long-term fitness goals effectively.

Understanding Periodization

Periodization divides training into specific periods or phases, each focusing on different aspects of fitness development:

Phases: Typically divided into macrocycles (annual plan), mesocycles (monthly or quarterly phases), and microcycles (weekly plans).

Goals: Aims to peak performance for specific events or competitions, optimize recovery, and promote continuous progress.

Example: Types of Periodization

Linear Periodization: Progressively increases intensity and decreases volume over time. Example: Starting with higher reps and lower weight in the hypertrophy phase, then transitioning to lower reps and higher weight in the strength phase.

Undulating Periodization: Varied intensity and volume within shorter periods (e.g., weekly or bi-weekly cycles). Example: Alternating between high volume and low volume workouts throughout the week to target different muscle fibers and metabolic pathways.

Benefits of Periodization

Progressive Adaptation: Allows for systematic progression and adaptation to training stimuli, optimizing muscle growth, strength gains, and endurance.

Injury Prevention: Balances workload and recovery periods, reducing the risk of overuse injuries associated with repetitive training.

Mental Refreshment: Provides mental variety and prevents training monotony, maintaining motivation and engagement.

Example: John's Periodization Plan

John incorporates linear periodization into his strength training program. He starts with a hypertrophy phase focusing on higher repetitions and moderate weights, gradually progressing to a strength phase with lower repetitions and heavier weights as he prepares for a powerlifting competition.

Implementing Periodization Techniques

Assessment and Planning: Assess current fitness level, set specific goals, and outline a periodized plan aligned with your objectives and timeline.

Phases and Cycles: Structure your training into distinct phases (e.g., hypertrophy, strength, power) and cycles (e.g., weekly, monthly) based on the desired outcomes.

Progression and Variation: Gradually increase intensity, adjust volume, and vary exercises to continuously challenge your body and promote adaptation.

Real-World Example: Sarah's Periodization Approach

Sarah incorporates undulating periodization into her marathon training program. She alternates between long-distance runs, speed workouts, and recovery days throughout the week, ensuring she develops both endurance and speed capabilities effectively.

Advanced Periodization Techniques

Peaking Phase: Fine-tunes training to optimize performance leading up to competitions or peak events, focusing on tapering and reducing training volume while maintaining intensity.

Deload Weeks: Periodic breaks or reduced training loads to facilitate recovery, prevent burnout, and allow for supercompensation (improved performance after recovery).

Example: Peak Phase for Powerlifting

Before a powerlifting competition, Jake incorporates a peaking phase into his training. He reduces training volume, maintains intensity with heavy lifts at competition weights, and focuses on perfecting technique and mental preparation.

Conclusion

Periodization techniques offer a structured approach to optimizing your workout program, enhancing performance, and achieving long-term fitness goals. By incorporating periodization principles such as linear, undulating, and peaking phases, you can tailor your training regimen to promote continuous progress, prevent plateauing, and sustain motivation throughout your fitness journey. In the following chapters, we'll explore advanced training methodologies, recovery strategies, and nutritional guidelines to further refine your workout program and help you achieve the perfect body with precision and efficiency.

Chapter 7: Designing An Effective Workout Program: Strength Training Essentials

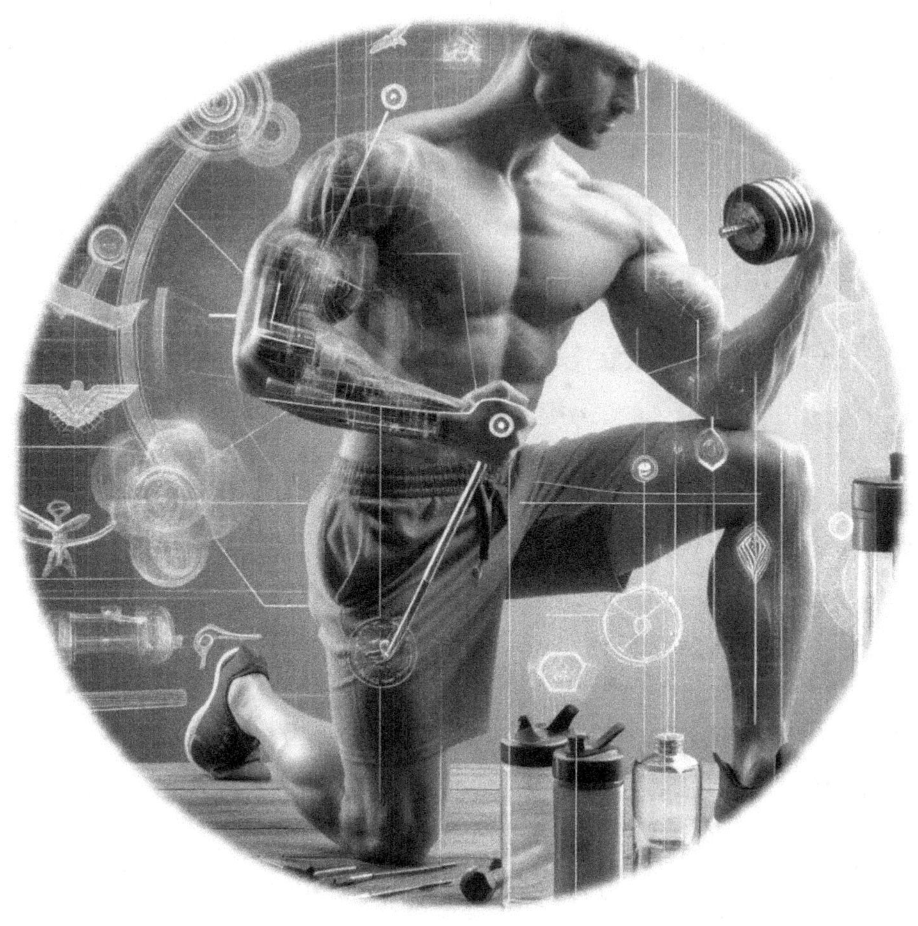

Core Exercises For Building Muscle

Core exercises play a fundamental role in strength training programs, providing stability, balance, and foundational strength essential for overall fitness and muscle development. This chapter explores key core exercises designed to build muscle and enhance functional strength, ensuring you achieve a well-rounded and effective workout regimen.

Importance of Core Strength

Core muscles, including the abdominals, obliques, lower back, and stabilizing muscles, contribute to:

Stability and Balance: Support proper posture and alignment during exercises and daily activities.

Strength and Power: Transfer force between the upper and lower body, crucial for lifting and athletic performance.

Injury Prevention: Protect the spine and surrounding structures from injury by maintaining stability and absorbing impact.

Example: Benefits of Core Strength

Developing core strength allows athletes like sprinters to maintain proper posture and stability during high-intensity sprints, reducing the risk of injuries and enhancing performance.

Key Core Exercises

Plank Variations: Engage the entire core, including the rectus abdominis, transverse abdominis, and obliques, promoting stability and endurance.

Example: Front Plank, Side Plank, Plank with Arm Lifts

Hanging Leg Raises: Target the lower abs and hip flexors, improving core strength and stability.

Example: Hanging Leg Raise with Knee Raises or Straight Leg Raises

Russian Twists: Activate the obliques and improve rotational strength and stability.

Example: Russian Twists with Medicine Ball or Dumbbell

Deadlifts: Strengthen the entire posterior chain, including the lower back and glutes, while improving core stability.

Example: Conventional Deadlifts, Sumo Deadlifts

Bridges: Activate the glutes and lower back muscles, enhancing core stability and hip strength.

Example: Glute Bridge, Single-Leg Bridge

Example Core Workout Routine

Warm-Up: 5-10 minutes of dynamic stretching and light cardio

Core Circuit (Perform each exercise for 3 sets of 12-15 reps):

Plank (Front Plank or Side Plank): 30 seconds hold each side

Hanging Leg Raises: 12 reps

Russian Twists (with Medicine Ball): 15 reps each side

Deadlifts: 3 sets x 8-10 reps

Bridges (Glute Bridge): 15 reps

Cool Down: 5-10 minutes of static stretching focusing on the core muscles

Integrating Core Exercises into Your Routine

Progression: Gradually increase the difficulty or intensity of core exercises by adding resistance, increasing repetitions, or incorporating unstable surfaces (e.g., stability balls, BOSU balls).

Variation: Rotate different core exercises to target various muscle groups and prevent plateauing.

Functional Application: Emphasize core stability during compound movements such as squats, deadlifts, and overhead presses to enhance overall strength and performance.

Real-World Example: Core Training for Endurance Athletes

Marathon runners incorporate core exercises like planks and bridges into their training regimen to improve running posture, maintain stability during long-distance runs, and reduce the risk of lower back injuries.

Conclusion

Incorporating core exercises into your strength training program is essential for developing overall strength, stability, and functional fitness. By performing a variety of core exercises targeting different muscle groups and integrating them strategically into your workout routine, you can enhance core strength, improve athletic performance, and reduce the risk of injuries. In the following chapters, we'll delve deeper into advanced strength training techniques, recovery strategies, and nutritional considerations to further optimize your workout program and help you achieve the perfect body with efficiency and precision.

Proper Form And Technique

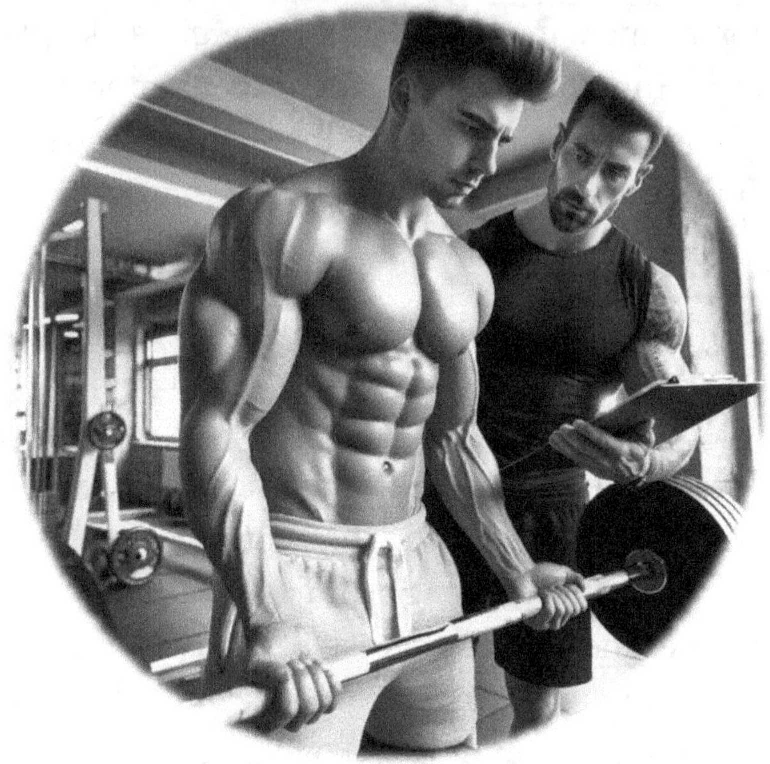

Mastering proper form and technique is crucial for maximizing the effectiveness of your strength training workouts while minimizing the risk of injuries. This chapter explores the importance of maintaining correct form during exercises, provides practical tips for achieving optimal technique, and highlights the benefits of prioritizing form in your fitness regimen.

Importance of Proper Form

Maintaining proper form and technique during strength training exercises offers several benefits:

Injury Prevention: Reduces the risk of strains, sprains, and other workout-related injuries by placing less stress on joints and muscles.

Muscle Activation: Ensures targeted muscles are properly engaged, optimizing muscle recruitment and promoting effective muscle growth.

Efficiency: Maximizes the efficiency of workouts by enhancing exercise effectiveness and minimizing wasted effort.

Example: Benefits of Proper Form

Using correct form during squats not only prevents lower back strain but also ensures proper activation of the quadriceps, hamstrings, and glutes, leading to improved strength gains and lower injury risk.

Principles of Proper Form and Technique

Alignment: Maintain proper body alignment throughout each exercise, ensuring joints are stacked and spine is neutral.

Range of Motion: Perform exercises through a full range of motion to maximize muscle activation and flexibility.

Controlled Movements: Avoid jerky or rapid movements; instead, focus on controlled, deliberate actions to maintain muscle tension.

Breathing: Coordinate your breathing with each movement, exhaling during the concentric (lifting) phase and inhaling during the eccentric (lowering) phase.

Tips for Achieving Proper Form

Start Light: Begin with lighter weights to practice and perfect your form before progressing to heavier loads.

Use Mirrors or Video: Utilize mirrors or record your workouts to visually assess your form and make necessary adjustments.

Engage Core Muscles: Activate your core muscles to stabilize your spine and maintain proper posture throughout exercises.

Seek Guidance: Consult with a certified trainer or fitness professional to learn proper techniques and receive feedback on your form.

Example: Squat Technique

Setup: Stand with feet shoulder-width apart, toes slightly turned out. Engage core, brace your abdominals.

Descent: Lower your body by bending at the knees and hips, keeping your chest up and back straight. Lower until thighs are parallel to the ground.

Ascent: Push through your heels, extend your knees and hips simultaneously, returning to the starting position.

Common Mistakes: Avoid leaning forward excessively, allowing knees to collapse inward, or lifting heels off the ground.

Real-World Application: Proper Deadlift Form

During deadlifts, maintain a flat back, hinge at the hips, and keep the barbell close to your body to reduce strain on your lower back and engage the glutes and hamstrings effectively.

Conclusion

Prioritizing proper form and technique in your strength training workouts is essential for maximizing results, preventing injuries, and enhancing overall fitness. By adhering to principles of alignment, range of motion, controlled movements, and proper breathing, you can optimize muscle activation and performance while minimizing the risk of overuse or strain. In the following chapters, we'll explore advanced strength training strategies, recovery techniques, and nutritional guidelines to further refine your workout program and help you achieve the perfect body with precision and safety.

Progressive Overload Strategies

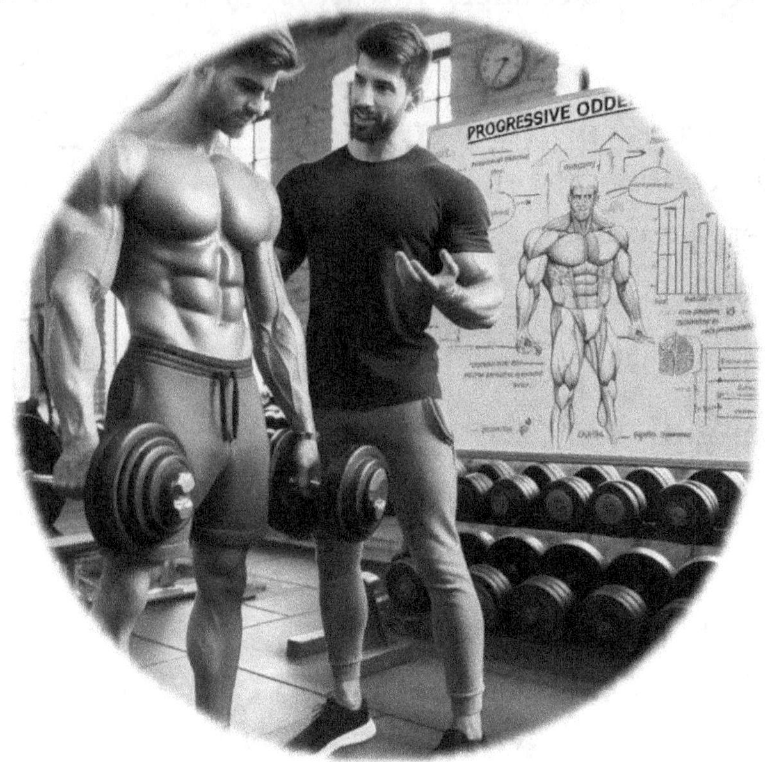

Progressive overload is a fundamental principle in strength training that involves gradually increasing the demands on your muscles to stimulate growth and adaptation. This chapter explores various progressive overload strategies, their benefits, and practical applications to help you achieve continuous improvements in strength and muscle development.

Understanding Progressive Overload

Progressive overload refers to the gradual increase in intensity, volume, or resistance of exercises over time to continually challenge the body and promote muscle growth. The principle is based on the concept that muscles must be subjected to increased stress to adapt and grow stronger.

Example: Benefits of Progressive Overload

By progressively increasing the weight lifted during bench presses, you force your muscles to adapt and grow stronger over time, leading to increased muscle mass and strength gains.

Progressive Overload Strategies

Increasing Resistance: Gradually increase the amount of weight lifted during exercises as your strength improves.

Example: Increase the weight on the barbell for squats by 5-10 pounds each week to challenge your muscles.

Adding Sets or Repetitions: Increase the number of sets or repetitions performed for each exercise to increase the overall workload.

Example: Perform 4 sets of 8-10 reps of shoulder presses instead of 3 sets to increase muscle endurance and strength.

Decreasing Rest Time: Shorten rest intervals between sets to maintain intensity and elevate heart rate, promoting muscle endurance and calorie burn.

Example: Reduce rest time from 60 seconds to 45 seconds between sets of push-ups to increase workout intensity.

Progressing Exercise Complexity: Advance to more challenging variations of exercises as you become proficient in basic movements.

Example: Progress from standard push-ups to decline push-ups or plyometric push-ups to increase upper body strength and explosive power.

Example: Progressive Overload in Deadlifts

Baseline: Start with a comfortable weight that allows you to perform 3 sets of 8 reps with good form.

Progression: Increase the weight by 5-10 pounds every 1-2 weeks, ensuring you can still complete the desired number of reps with proper technique.

Outcome: Over time, your muscles adapt to the increased demand, leading to improved strength and muscle development.

Practical Applications of Progressive Overload

Tracking Progress: Keep a workout journal or use a fitness app to record sets, reps, and weights used for each exercise, allowing you to monitor progress and adjust accordingly.

Periodization: Incorporate progressive overload into structured training phases (e.g., hypertrophy, strength, power) to optimize muscle adaptation and prevent plateaus.

Listen to Your Body: Gradually increase intensity and volume while listening to your body's feedback to avoid overtraining and injuries.

Real-World Example: Strength Training Program

John incorporates progressive overload into his strength training program by increasing resistance and varying exercises every 4-6 weeks to continually challenge his muscles and avoid stagnation.

Conclusion

Progressive overload is a cornerstone principle in strength training that promotes consistent improvements in muscle strength, size, and endurance. By strategically increasing resistance, volume, or intensity over time, you can stimulate muscle growth and adaptation effectively while minimizing the risk of overuse injuries. In the following chapters, we'll explore advanced strength training methodologies, recovery strategies, and nutritional considerations to further enhance your workout program and help you achieve the perfect body with precision and sustainable progress.

Chapter 8: Advanced Muscle-Building Techniques

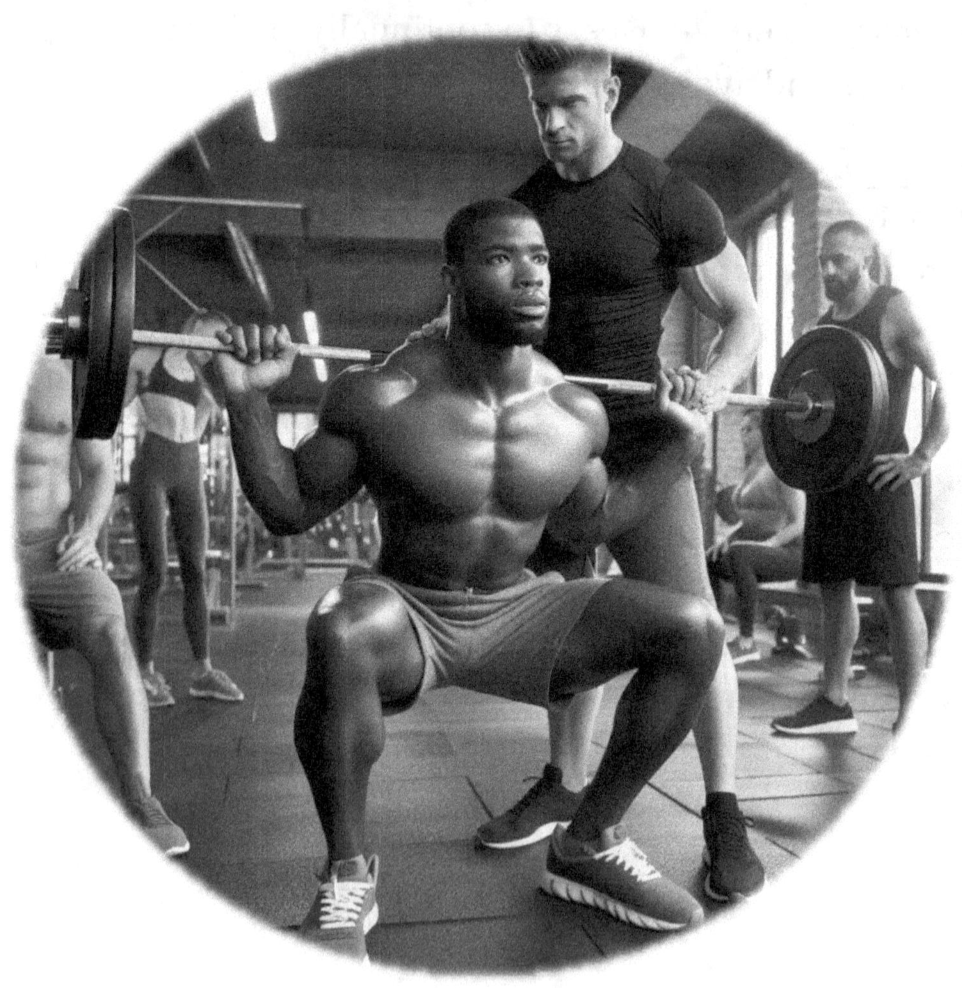

Supersets, Drop Sets, And Pyramid Sets

Advanced muscle-building techniques such as supersets, drop sets, and pyramid sets are powerful strategies used to intensify workouts, promote muscle hypertrophy, and enhance overall muscular endurance. This chapter delves into each technique, explores their benefits, and provides practical examples to incorporate them into your training regimen effectively.

Understanding Advanced Muscle-Building Techniques

These techniques manipulate various aspects of training intensity and volume to challenge muscles in unique ways, stimulating greater muscle fiber recruitment and metabolic stress for enhanced growth and conditioning.

Supersets: Maximizing Efficiency and Intensity

Supersets involve performing two exercises back-to-back with minimal rest between sets, targeting either the same muscle group (agonist superset) or opposing muscle groups (antagonist superset).

Example: Pairing bench presses (chest) with bent-over rows (back) in an antagonistic superset to maximize upper body pump and efficiency.

Drop Sets: Pushing Muscular Endurance to the Limit

Drop sets involve performing a set to failure, then immediately reducing the weight and continuing with another set without rest. This technique challenges muscles to perform additional reps beyond fatigue, promoting metabolic stress and muscle hypertrophy.

Example: Performing bicep curls with a heavy weight until failure, then immediately switching to a lighter weight to continue curls until failure again.

Pyramid Sets: Progressive Overload in Action

Pyramid sets involve gradually increasing or decreasing the weight and/or reps with each set. This technique allows for progressive overload within a single exercise, stimulating muscle fibers across different intensity levels.

Example: Performing bench presses starting with lighter weights and higher reps, then increasing weight and decreasing reps with each subsequent set.

Benefits of Advanced Muscle-Building Techniques

Increased Muscle Hypertrophy: Stimulate muscle growth through increased time under tension and metabolic stress.

Enhanced Muscular Endurance: Improve muscle stamina and resistance to fatigue, crucial for prolonged athletic performance.

Time Efficiency: Maximize workout efficiency by targeting multiple muscle groups or intensifying training volume within a shorter period.

Example: Real-World Application

Sarah incorporates drop sets into her leg workout routine by performing squats with a challenging weight until failure, then reducing the weight and continuing to squat until reaching muscle fatigue, effectively enhancing lower body strength and endurance.

Practical Tips for Implementing Advanced Techniques

Progress Gradually: Introduce these techniques gradually into your routine to allow your body to adapt and minimize injury risk.

Monitor Intensity: Adjust weight and volume based on your fitness level and goals to ensure proper form and avoid overtraining.

Variation: Rotate different advanced techniques periodically to prevent plateauing and maintain workout motivation.

Example: Superset Routine for Upper Body

Superset 1:

Bench Press (4 sets x 8-10 reps)

Bent-over Rows (4 sets x 8-10 reps)

<u>**Superset 2:**</u>
Overhead Shoulder Press (3 sets x 10-12 reps)

Pull-ups (3 sets x max reps)

<u>Conclusion</u>

Incorporating supersets, drop sets, and pyramid sets into your workout regimen can significantly enhance muscle growth, strength, and endurance by manipulating training variables to create new challenges for your muscles. These advanced techniques provide versatility and intensity, making them valuable additions to any comprehensive strength training program. In the following chapters, we'll explore advanced training methodologies, recovery strategies, and nutritional guidelines to further optimize your workout program and help you achieve the perfect body with precision and sustainable progress.

Time Under Tension

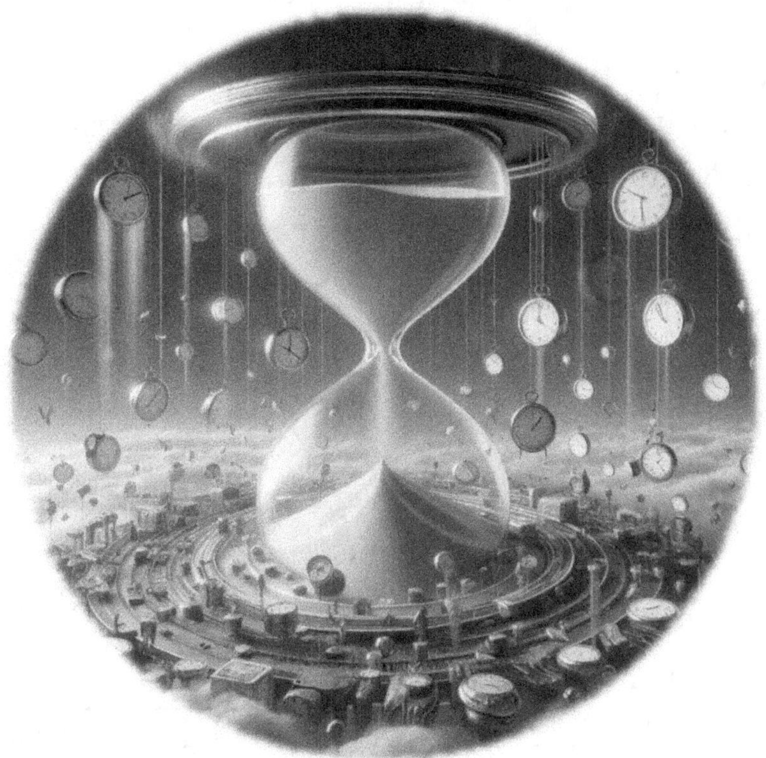

Time under tension (TUT) is a crucial concept in strength training that focuses on prolonging the duration muscles are under strain during exercises. This chapter explores the significance of TUT in muscle hypertrophy, practical applications of this technique, and how to incorporate it effectively into your workout routine to achieve optimal results.

Understanding Time Under Tension

Time under tension refers to the amount of time muscles are actively engaged during each repetition of an exercise. By manipulating the tempo of movements and controlling the speed of each phase (concentric, eccentric, and isometric), you can increase muscle fiber recruitment and metabolic stress, both essential for muscle growth.

Benefits of Time Under Tension

Increased Muscle Hypertrophy: Prolonged tension on muscles promotes micro-tears in muscle fibers, stimulating growth and adaptation.

Enhanced Muscle Endurance: Improves muscular stamina and resistance to fatigue by challenging muscles through extended time under load.

Improved Mind-Muscle Connection: Heightens awareness and control over muscle contractions, optimizing exercise effectiveness and muscle activation.

Example: Benefits of Slow Eccentric Movements

Performing slow eccentric (lowering) phases during exercises like squats or bicep curls increases time under tension, leading to greater muscle fiber recruitment and enhancing strength gains.

Practical Applications of Time Under Tension

Tempo Manipulation: Control the speed of each phase of an exercise (e.g., 2 seconds concentric, 4 seconds eccentric) to maximize muscle engagement and metabolic stress.

Isometric Holds: Integrate pauses or holds at the midpoint or end range of motion to increase time under tension and challenge muscle endurance.

Drop Sets with TUT: Combine drop sets (reducing weight after failure) with extended time under tension to exhaust muscle fibers and stimulate hypertrophy.

Example: Squat with Increased Time Under Tension

Setup: Begin with feet shoulder-width apart, holding a barbell across your upper back.

Execution: Lower into a squat position, taking 3-4 seconds to descend (eccentric phase), pause for 1-2 seconds at the bottom (isometric phase), then explode upward for 1-2 seconds (concentric phase).

Repetition: Repeat for 8-12 reps, focusing on maintaining control and tension throughout each phase of the movement.

Real-World Application: TUT in Bodyweight Exercises

Performing push-ups with a slow and controlled descent (eccentric phase) followed by a brief pause at the bottom enhances time under tension, promoting chest and triceps development effectively.

Incorporating Time Under Tension into Your Workout Routine

Focus on Form: Prioritize proper technique and form to maximize muscle engagement and minimize injury risk.

Progressive Overload: Gradually increase the duration of time under tension or resistance to continually challenge muscles and induce adaptation.

Variety: Rotate exercises and tempos regularly to prevent adaptation and stimulate continuous muscle growth.

Example: TUT Routine for Upper Body
Exercise 1: Bench Press
Tempo: 3 seconds down (eccentric), 1-second pause (isometric), 2 seconds up (concentric)

Sets/Reps: 4 sets x 8-10 reps

Exercise 2: Bicep Curls
Tempo: 2 seconds up (concentric), 4 seconds down (eccentric)

Sets/Reps: 3 sets x 12-15 reps

Conclusion
Time under tension is a potent technique in strength training that enhances muscle hypertrophy, endurance, and overall workout effectiveness. By deliberately controlling the tempo of exercises and extending the duration muscles are under strain, you can optimize muscle growth and development. In the following chapters, we'll explore additional advanced training methodologies, recovery strategies, and nutritional considerations to further refine your workout program and help you achieve the perfect body with precision and sustainable progress.

Incorporating Variety Into Your Workouts

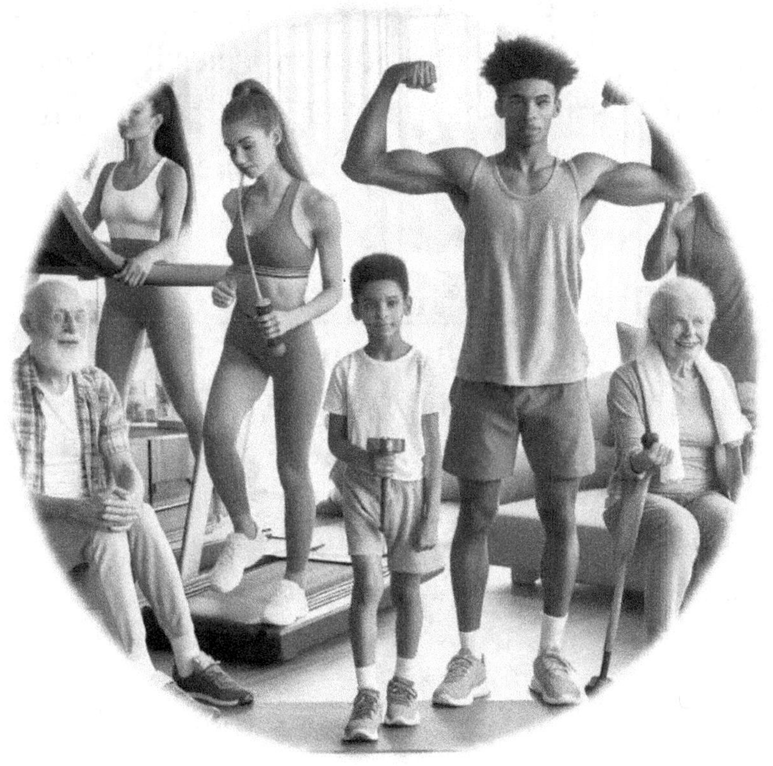

Variety is not just the spice of life but also the key to achieving continuous progress in your fitness journey. This chapter explores the importance of incorporating variety into your workouts, provides examples of different methods, and discusses how diverse training approaches can optimize muscle building and prevent training plateaus.

Understanding the Role of Variety

Variety in workouts refers to the systematic inclusion of different exercises, training methods, and variables such as intensity, volume, and tempo. By regularly changing these aspects, you challenge your muscles in new ways, stimulate different muscle fibers, and prevent your body from adapting to a specific routine, which can lead to plateaus.

Benefits of Incorporating Variety

Muscle Confusion: Introducing new exercises and training methods keeps muscles guessing and promotes continual adaptation and growth.

Prevention of Plateaus: Avoid stagnation and boredom by continuously challenging muscles with diverse workouts, leading to sustained progress.

Injury Prevention: Varying exercises reduces the risk of overuse injuries by distributing stress across different muscle groups and movement patterns.

Example: Benefits of Workout Variation

Incorporating resistance bands into your routine alongside free weights challenges stabilizing muscles and improves joint mobility, enhancing overall functional strength and flexibility.

Practical Strategies for Workout Variety

Exercise Selection: Rotate between compound and isolation exercises to target different muscle groups and movement patterns.

Training Modalities: Alternate between strength training, cardiovascular exercises, flexibility work, and functional movements to maintain overall fitness.

Intensity Techniques: Integrate techniques such as supersets, drop sets, and pyramid sets to vary workout intensity and stimulate muscle growth.

Example: Sample Weekly Workout Schedule

Monday: Strength Training (Compound Movements)

Squats, Deadlifts, Bench Press

Wednesday: Cardiovascular Training

Running, Cycling, or HIIT

Friday: Functional Training

Bodyweight exercises, Core work, Stability exercises

Incorporating Periodization for Long-Term Success

Periodization involves dividing your training into specific phases (e.g., hypertrophy, strength, power) with varying intensities and goals. This structured approach not only prevents overtraining but also optimizes performance and muscle development over time.

Example: Periodized Training Program

Phase 1: Hypertrophy

Focus on moderate to high reps and volume to stimulate muscle growth.

Phase 2: Strength

Increase intensity with lower reps and heavier weights to build foundational strength.

Phase 3: Power

Emphasize explosive movements and plyometrics to enhance speed and power output.

Real-World Application: Workout Variation for Muscle Definition

Incorporate yoga or Pilates sessions alongside weightlifting to improve flexibility, core strength, and muscle definition, enhancing overall physique and athletic performance.

Conclusion

Incorporating variety into your workouts is essential for optimizing muscle growth, preventing plateaus, and maintaining long-term fitness progress. By diversifying exercises, training methods, and intensity levels, you can challenge your body in new ways, stimulate muscle adaptation, and achieve balanced muscular development. In the following chapters, we'll delve deeper into advanced training methodologies, recovery techniques, and nutritional strategies to further refine your workout program and help you achieve the perfect body with precision and sustainable progress.

Chapter 9: Nutrition Strategies For Muscle Gain

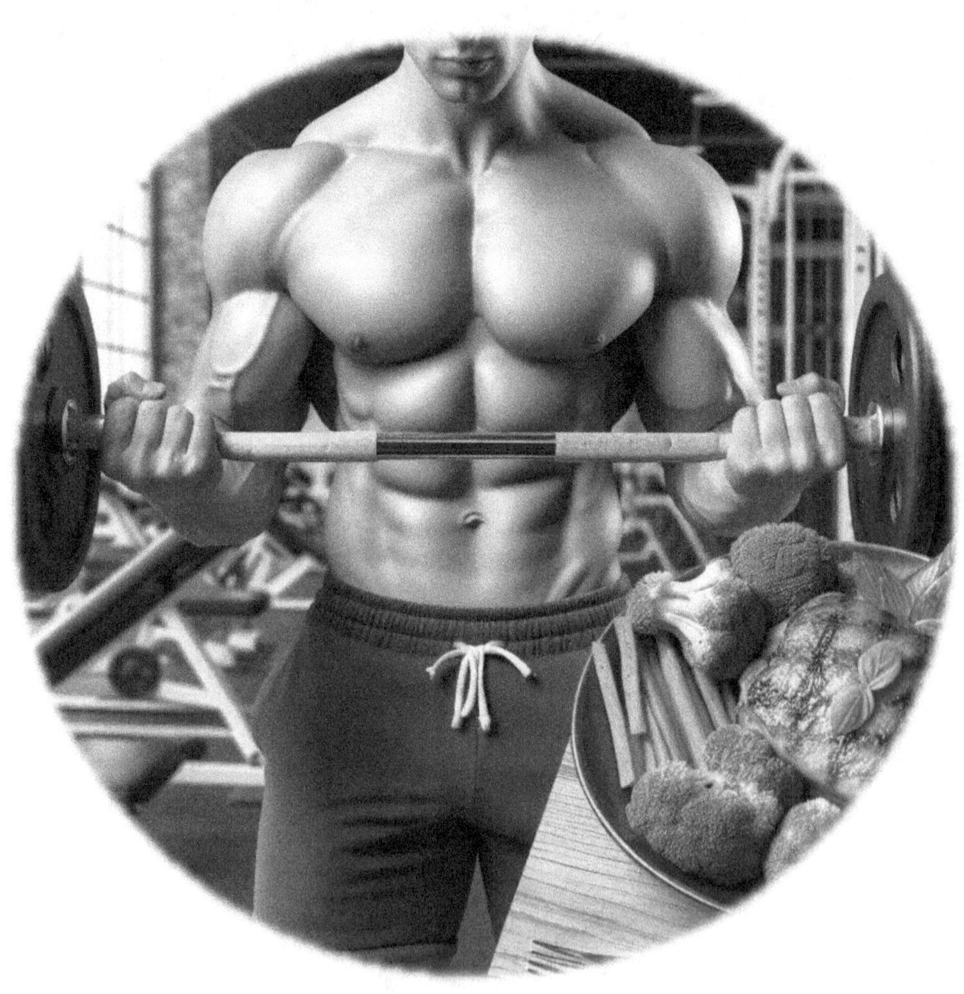

Pre- And Post-Workout Nutrition

Nutrition plays a pivotal role in supporting muscle growth, enhancing performance, and accelerating recovery. This chapter focuses on the importance of pre- and post-workout nutrition, provides practical strategies, and discusses how timing and nutrient composition can maximize your training results.

Understanding Pre-Workout Nutrition

Pre-workout nutrition involves consuming the right nutrients at the right time to prepare your body for exercise, optimize performance, and minimize muscle breakdown. The goal is to provide energy, enhance focus, and promote muscle protein synthesis.

Components of Effective Pre-Workout Nutrition

Carbohydrates: Provide readily available energy to fuel muscles during exercise.

Example: Whole grain toast with peanut butter provides complex carbs and protein for sustained energy.

Protein: Supports muscle repair and growth, especially when combined with carbohydrates.

Example: Greek yogurt with berries offers a blend of protein and carbs ideal for pre-workout fuel.

Hydration: Ensures optimal fluid balance and helps maintain exercise performance.

Example: Drink 8-16 ounces of water or a sports drink 1-2 hours before exercise to stay hydrated.

Example: Pre-Workout Meal

Meal Idea: Grilled chicken breast with sweet potatoes and steamed vegetables provides a balanced combination of protein, complex carbohydrates, and vitamins to fuel intense workouts.

Timing Pre-Workout Nutrition

Consuming a balanced meal or snack containing carbs and protein 1-3 hours before exercise allows adequate digestion and absorption, optimizing nutrient availability during workouts.

Understanding Post-Workout Nutrition

Post-workout nutrition is crucial for replenishing glycogen stores, repairing muscle tissue, and promoting muscle protein synthesis. Timing and nutrient composition play key roles in enhancing recovery and supporting muscle growth.

Components of Effective Post-Workout Nutrition

Protein: Essential for muscle repair and growth.

Example: Whey protein shake or lean protein source like grilled chicken or tofu.

Carbohydrates: Replenishes glycogen stores and enhances recovery.

Example: Brown rice or quinoa combined with a lean protein source provides carbs and amino acids for recovery.

Fluids and Electrolytes: Rehydrate to replace fluids lost through sweat and maintain electrolyte balance.

Example: Coconut water or a sports drink helps replenish electrolytes post-exercise.

Example: Post-Workout Snack

Snack Idea: Banana with almond butter provides carbs for glycogen replenishment and protein for muscle repair, ideal within 30 minutes after exercise.

Nutrient Timing for Optimal Recovery

Consuming a combination of protein and carbs within 30-60 minutes post-exercise enhances muscle glycogen replenishment and promotes muscle repair and growth.

Real-World Application: Post-Workout Nutrition Routine

Ella incorporates a protein shake with banana immediately after her strength training sessions to facilitate muscle recovery and replenish energy stores effectively.

<u>Conclusion</u>

Optimizing pre- and post-workout nutrition is essential for maximizing muscle gain, enhancing performance, and accelerating recovery. By strategically timing nutrient intake and choosing nutrient-dense foods, you can support muscle protein synthesis, replenish energy stores, and promote overall fitness progress. In the following chapters, we'll explore advanced nutrition strategies, supplementation tips, and meal planning techniques to further refine your nutrition approach and help you achieve the perfect body with precision and sustainable progress.

Importance Of Protein Intake

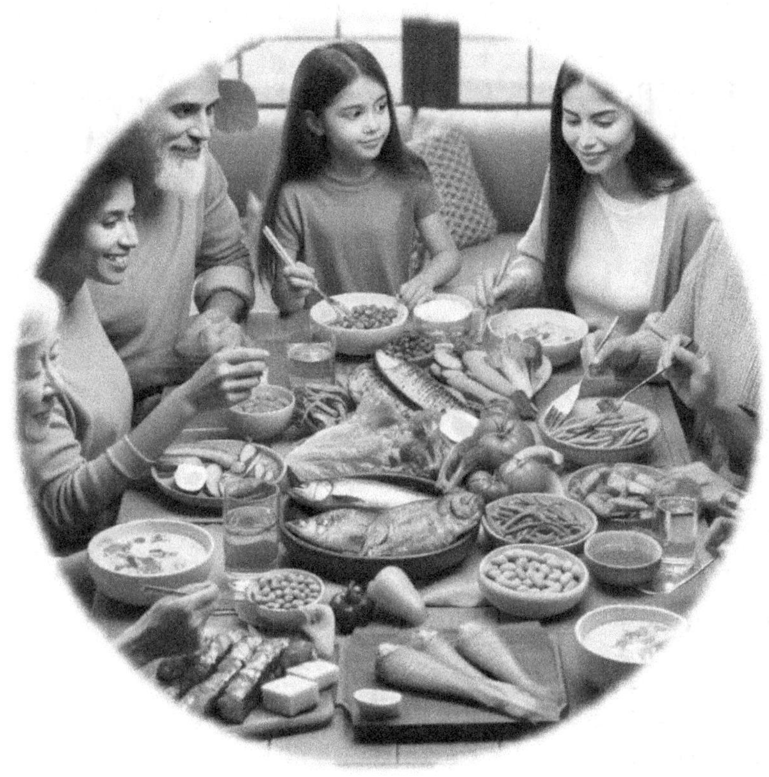

Protein is a crucial macronutrient essential for muscle growth, repair, and maintenance. Its role in supporting muscle gain cannot be overstated, making it a cornerstone of any effective muscle-building nutrition plan.

Protein's Role in Muscle Gain

Muscle Repair and Growth: Protein provides the building blocks (amino acids) necessary for repairing and building muscle tissue damaged during exercise.

Muscle Protein Synthesis: Consuming adequate protein stimulates muscle protein synthesis, the process by which muscles repair and grow larger in response to training.

Metabolic Functions: Protein plays roles in various metabolic processes, including enzyme production, hormone regulation, and immune function.

Protein Requirements for Muscle Gain

Daily Intake: Aim for 0.7 to 1 gram of protein per pound of body weight per day, depending on activity level and training intensity.

Timing: Distribute protein intake evenly throughout the day, including pre- and post-workout meals/snacks to optimize muscle recovery and growth.

Sources of High-Quality Protein

Animal Sources: Lean meats (chicken, turkey, beef), fish, eggs, and dairy products (milk, yogurt).

Plant Sources: Legumes (beans, lentils), tofu, tempeh, quinoa, nuts, and seeds.

Example: Protein-Rich Meal Ideas

Breakfast: Greek yogurt with berries and nuts.

Lunch: Grilled chicken breast with quinoa and vegetables.

Snack: Cottage cheese with fruit.

Dinner: Salmon with sweet potatoes and steamed broccoli.

Real-World Application: Protein Timing and Muscle Gain

Consuming a protein-rich snack such as a protein shake or a chicken breast after a workout helps replenish amino acids and promotes muscle repair and growth.

Conclusion

Protein intake is foundational for muscle gain, supporting muscle repair, growth, and overall metabolic health. By ensuring adequate daily intake and strategic timing around workouts, you can optimize muscle protein synthesis and achieve your muscle-building goals effectively. In the following chapters, we'll delve deeper into advanced nutrition strategies, supplementation tips, and practical meal planning to further refine your approach and help you achieve the perfect body with sustainable progress.

Supplements For Muscle Growth

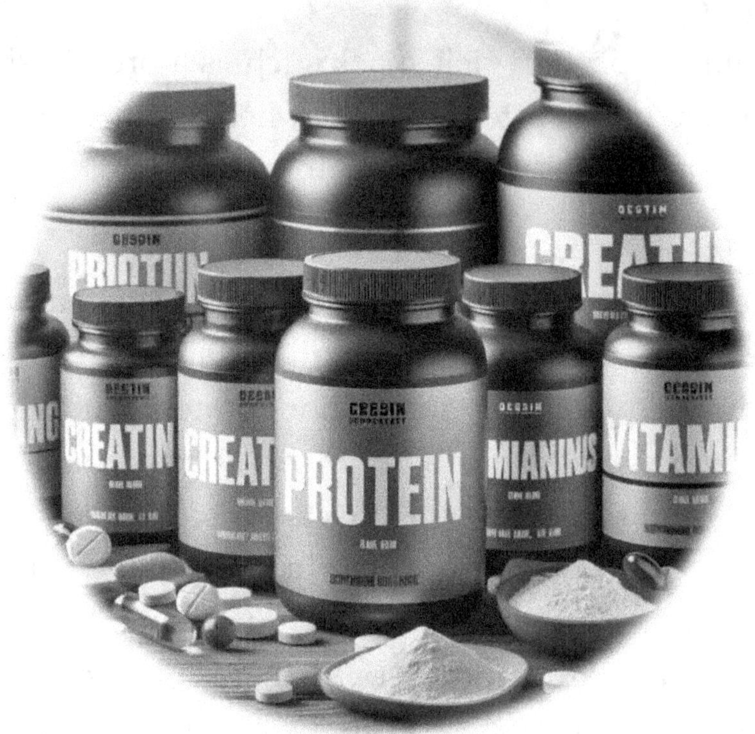

Supplements play a supportive role in muscle gain by providing additional nutrients that may be challenging to obtain solely through diet. This chapter explores popular supplements for muscle growth, their benefits, and considerations for incorporating them into your nutrition regimen.

Understanding Supplements for Muscle Growth

Supplements are products intended to complement a balanced diet and support overall health and performance goals. When used strategically and in conjunction with a nutritious diet and proper training program, certain supplements can enhance muscle recovery, promote muscle protein synthesis, and optimize performance.

Popular Supplements for Muscle Growth

Whey Protein: A fast-digesting protein source that supports muscle repair and growth, ideal for post-workout recovery.

Example: Mixing whey protein powder with water or milk provides a convenient post-workout protein boost.

Creatine: Enhances ATP production, improving strength and power output during high-intensity exercise.

Example: Taking 5 grams of creatine monohydrate daily can increase muscle creatine stores over time, supporting performance in strength training.

Branched-Chain Amino Acids (BCAAs): Leucine, isoleucine, and valine aid in muscle protein synthesis and reduce muscle breakdown.

Example: Consuming BCAAs before or during workouts can support muscle recovery and reduce exercise-induced muscle damage.

Beta-Alanine: Increases muscle carnosine levels, buffering acidity in muscles during intense exercise, delaying fatigue.

Example: Taking beta-alanine supplements may improve performance in high-intensity activities like sprinting or weightlifting.

Example: Supplement Timing and Usage

Timing: Incorporate whey protein within 30 minutes post-workout to enhance muscle recovery and protein synthesis.

Usage: Cycling creatine supplements with loading and maintenance phases can optimize muscle creatine stores for enhanced performance.

Considerations for Supplement Use

Quality: Choose reputable brands with third-party testing to ensure purity and quality of supplements.

Dosage: Follow recommended dosages and guidelines provided by manufacturers or healthcare professionals.

Individual Needs: Consider individual factors such as training intensity, diet, and health conditions when selecting supplements.

Real-World Application: Integrating Supplements into Your Routine

John includes a whey protein shake after his strength training sessions to support muscle recovery and growth, while also taking creatine to enhance his performance during workouts.

Conclusion

Supplements can be valuable tools for enhancing muscle growth and performance when used judiciously alongside a well-balanced diet and structured training program. Understanding the benefits and considerations of each supplement allows you to make informed choices that align with your fitness goals. In the following chapters, we'll continue to explore advanced nutrition strategies, meal planning techniques, and holistic approaches to help you achieve the perfect body with sustainable progress.

Chapter 10: Overcoming Plateaus

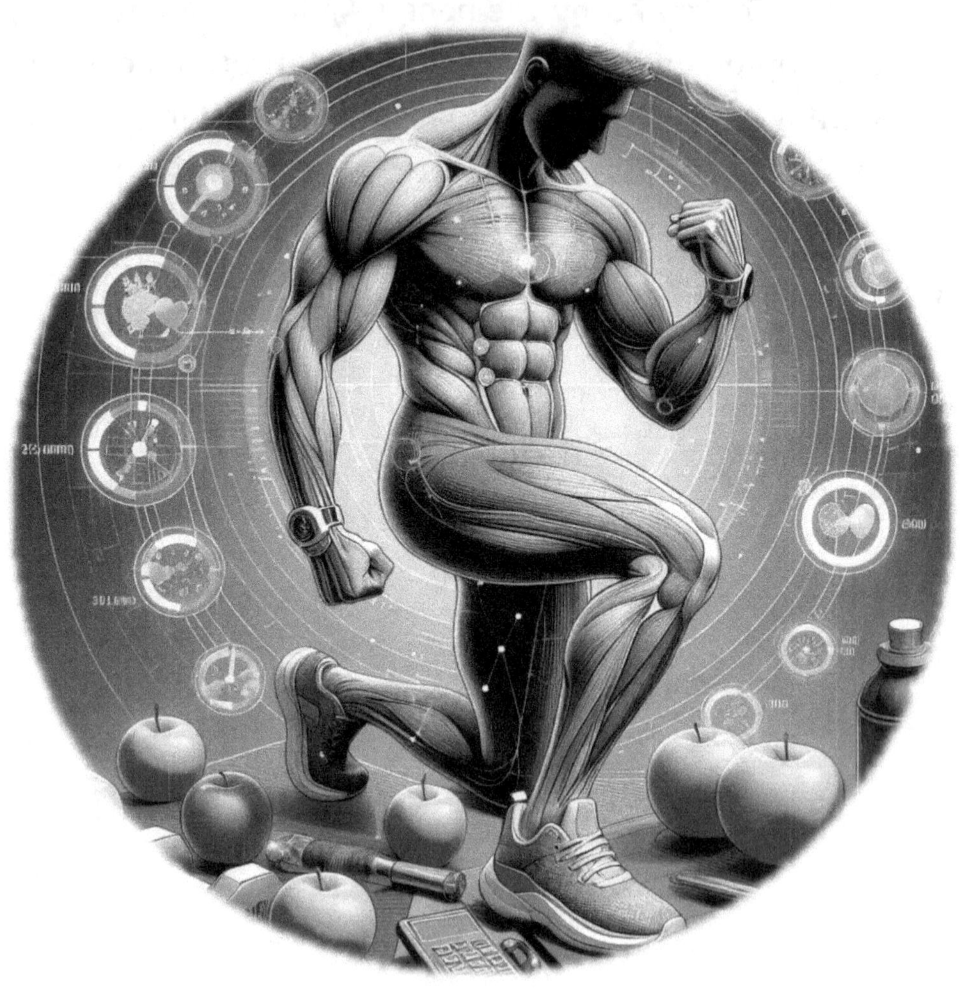

Identifying And Addressing Stagnation

Plateaus are common in any fitness regimen and can be frustrating. This chapter explores strategies to identify and overcome plateaus, ensuring continual progress towards your fitness goals.

Recognizing Signs of Plateaus

Lack of Progress: Stagnant or minimal improvements in strength, muscle mass, or endurance despite consistent effort.

Decreased Motivation: Feeling unmotivated or disinterested in workouts due to lack of visible results.

Physical and Mental Fatigue: Persistent tiredness or feeling drained during and after workouts.

Causes of Plateaus

Overtraining: Insufficient recovery time between workouts leading to diminished performance.

Routine Consistency: Sticking to the same exercises, intensity, and volume without variation.

Nutritional Deficiencies: Inadequate intake of nutrients crucial for muscle repair and growth.

Strategies to Overcome Plateaus

Modify Your Workout Routine: Introduce new exercises, change intensity levels, or incorporate different training modalities like HIIT or circuit training.

Adjust Nutrition: Ensure adequate protein intake, consider nutrient timing around workouts, and evaluate overall caloric intake to support energy needs.

Optimize Recovery: Prioritize sleep, incorporate active recovery techniques like yoga or light cardio, and consider rest days to allow muscles adequate time to repair and grow.

Example: Breaking Through a Strength Plateau

If you've hit a plateau in your bench press strength:

Variation: Incorporate incline or decline bench presses to target different angles of the chest.

Intensity: Adjust weights and rep ranges to challenge your muscles differently.

Form: Ensure proper form and technique to maximize muscle engagement and prevent injury.

Real-World Application: Tracking Progress and Adjustments

Jenna keeps a workout journal to track her lifts, noting when she hits a plateau. She adjusts her routine by increasing weights gradually and varying her exercises to stimulate muscle growth effectively.

Conclusion

Identifying and addressing plateaus is essential for maintaining progress in your fitness journey. By recognizing signs of stagnation, implementing strategic changes to your workout routine, and optimizing recovery and nutrition, you can overcome plateaus and continue making strides towards achieving your fitness goals. In the following chapters, we'll explore advanced training methodologies, nutrition strategies, and lifestyle adjustments to further support your pursuit of the perfect body with sustainable progress.

Adjusting Workout Intensity And Volume

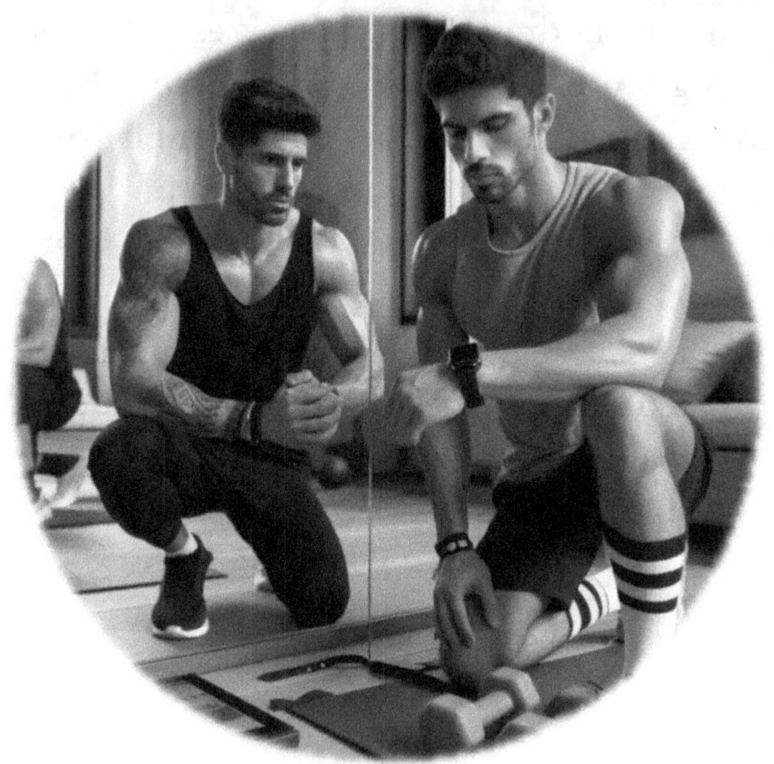

Plateaus in fitness progress can often be overcome by strategically adjusting the intensity and volume of your workouts. This chapter delves into effective methods to adjust these variables to reignite progress and achieve new levels of fitness.

Understanding Workout Intensity and Volume

Workout Intensity: Refers to the level of effort exerted during exercise, often measured by weight, repetitions, or perceived exertion.

Workout Volume: Represents the total amount of work performed in a single session, typically calculated by sets, reps, and weight lifted.

Signs of Plateaus in Intensity and Volume

Stagnant Progress: No noticeable improvements in strength, endurance, or muscle growth despite consistent training.

Decreased Performance: Inability to lift heavier weights or complete workouts with previous intensity.

Strategies to Adjust Intensity and Volume

Progressive Overload: Gradually increase the weight lifted to challenge muscles and stimulate growth.

Example: Increase the weight by 5-10% for compound lifts like squats or deadlifts to push beyond current limits.

Variation in Repetitions: Modify rep ranges (e.g., lower reps with heavier weights or higher reps with lighter weights) to target different muscle fibers and break monotony.

Example: Alternate between 3-5 reps for strength and 8-12 reps for hypertrophy during different phases of training.

Periodization: Implement structured periods of high and low intensity/volume to prevent overtraining and promote recovery.

Example: Incorporate deload weeks every 4-6 weeks, reducing volume and intensity to allow for physiological and psychological recovery.

Example: Adjusting Workout Intensity

If you're plateauing in your squat strength:
Intensity: Increase weight incrementally over several weeks to challenge your muscles.

Volume: Adjust sets and reps to optimize muscle fatigue without compromising form.

Real-World Application: Tracking Progress and Adjustments
Tom monitors his workout performance using a fitness app, noting when he reaches a plateau. He adjusts his training plan by progressively increasing weights and varying rep ranges to stimulate muscle growth effectively.

Conclusion
Adjusting workout intensity and volume is key to overcoming plateaus and achieving continuous progress in your fitness journey. By strategically modifying these variables, incorporating progressive overload principles, and implementing periodization techniques, you can break through barriers and reach new levels of strength, endurance, and muscle growth. In the following chapters, we'll explore advanced training methodologies, nutrition

strategies, and holistic approaches to support your pursuit of the perfect body with sustainable progress.

Psychological Strategies To Stay Motivated

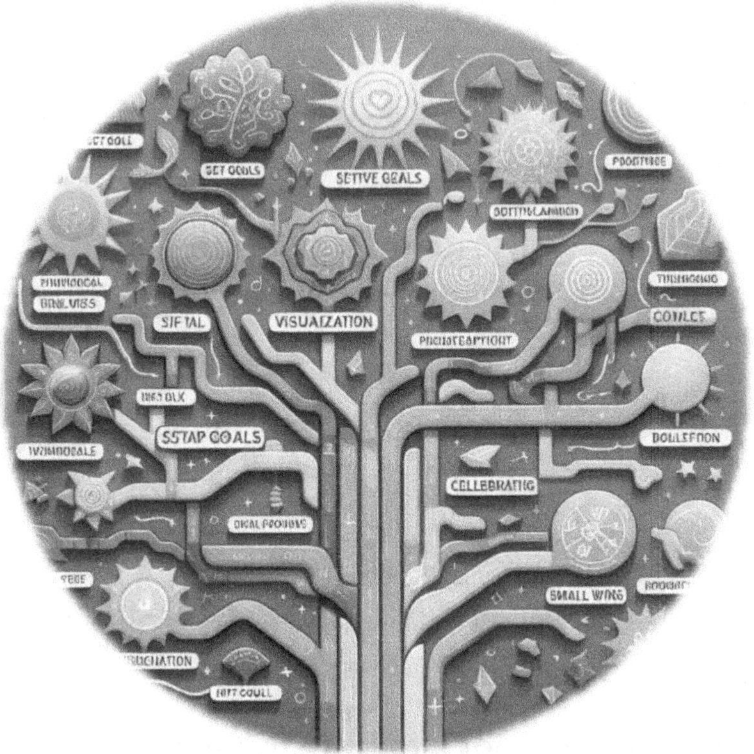

Overcoming plateaus in fitness often requires not just physical adjustments but also psychological strategies to sustain motivation and continue making progress. This chapter explores effective methods to stay motivated and mentally resilient during challenging phases of your fitness journey.

Understanding Motivation in Fitness

Intrinsic vs. Extrinsic Motivation: Intrinsic motivation comes from within, driven by personal enjoyment or satisfaction (e.g., feeling good after a workout). Extrinsic motivation stems from external rewards or recognition (e.g., winning a competition).

Goal Setting: Setting specific, measurable, attainable, relevant, and time-bound (SMART) goals helps maintain focus and direction.

Common Psychological Challenges

Loss of Interest: Feeling bored or uninspired with workouts.

Frustration: Experiencing setbacks or not seeing immediate results.

Strategies to Stay Motivated

Visualize Success: Imagine achieving your fitness goals and how it will positively impact your life.

Example: Create a vision board with images of your ideal physique or fitness achievements to stay inspired.

Celebrate Milestones: Acknowledge and celebrate small achievements along the way to keep motivation high.

Example: Treat yourself to a massage or a healthy meal after reaching a new personal record in lifting.

Find Social Support: Surround yourself with supportive friends, workout buddies, or join fitness communities to stay motivated.

Example: Participate in group fitness classes or online fitness challenges to stay connected and motivated.

Example: Overcoming Psychological Plateaus

If you're struggling with motivation during a plateau:

Reassess Goals: Reflect on why you started your fitness journey and adjust goals if necessary to stay aligned with your values and aspirations.

Change Your Routine: Try new exercises or workout formats to add variety and excitement to your workouts.

Real-World Application: Building Mental Resilience

Sara uses positive self-talk during challenging workouts to stay motivated and focused. She reminds herself of her progress and visualizes achieving her fitness goals to maintain momentum.

Conclusion

Psychological strategies play a crucial role in overcoming plateaus and sustaining long-term fitness progress. By understanding your motivations, setting meaningful goals, and implementing strategies to stay resilient during setbacks, you can navigate challenges effectively and continue moving forward in your fitness journey. In the following chapters, we'll explore advanced training methodologies, nutrition strategies, and holistic approaches to support your pursuit of the perfect body with sustainable progress.

Conclusion

Congratulations on completing this journey towards building the perfect body and enhancing your physical performance! Throughout this ebook, we've explored a wide range of topics designed to empower you with the knowledge and strategies necessary for achieving your fitness goals. Let's recap some of the key points covered in each section:

Chapter Summaries

The Science of Muscle Growth

Understanding muscle hypertrophy and the importance of progressive overload.

Example: "By progressively increasing the weight you lift over time, you stimulate muscle fibers to adapt and grow stronger."

The Physiology of Fat Loss

Exploring metabolic processes and hormonal influences on fat metabolism.

Example: "Hormones like insulin and cortisol play crucial roles in fat storage and breakdown, impacting our ability to lose fat effectively."

Nutrition Fundamentals

Discussing macronutrients, micronutrients, and calculating caloric needs.

Example: "Proper nutrition ensures you have the energy and nutrients necessary for optimal performance and recovery."

The Importance of Rest and Recovery

Highlighting sleep, active vs. passive recovery, and the role of rest days.

Example: "Quality sleep promotes muscle repair and growth, while strategic rest days prevent overtraining and reduce injury risk."

Setting Realistic Goals

Using SMART criteria for goal-setting and tracking progress.

Example: "Setting specific, measurable, attainable, relevant, and time-bound goals helps maintain motivation and focus."

Designing an Effective Workout Program

Comparing split routines vs. full-body workouts and discussing periodization techniques.

Example: "Periodization allows for systematic variation in intensity and volume to prevent plateaus and optimize progress."

Strength Training Essentials

Focusing on core exercises, proper form, and progressive overload strategies.

Example: "Mastering proper form ensures you maximize muscle engagement and minimize injury risk during strength training."

Advanced Muscle-Building Techniques

Exploring supersets, drop sets, pyramid sets, time under tension, and incorporating variety.

Example: "Variety in training keeps workouts engaging and challenges muscles in new ways, promoting continuous growth."

Nutrition Strategies for Muscle Gain

Emphasizing protein intake, supplements, and dietary strategies for muscle growth.

Example: "Protein is crucial for muscle repair and growth, making it essential to consume adequate amounts throughout the day."

Overcoming Plateaus

Adjusting workout intensity and volume and using psychological strategies for motivation.

Example: "Changing workout variables and staying mentally resilient are key to overcoming plateaus and continuing progress."

Recap of Key Insights

Understanding Muscle Growth and Fat Loss: We delved into the science behind muscle hypertrophy and effective fat loss strategies, emphasizing the importance of nutrition and training.

Nutrition Fundamentals: Exploring the role of macronutrients, micronutrients, and calculating caloric needs for optimal performance and recovery.

Rest and Recovery: Highlighting the critical role of sleep, active recovery, and rest days in preventing overtraining and promoting muscle repair.

Goal Setting and Progress Tracking: Using SMART goals to maintain motivation and tracking progress to adjust training and nutrition plans effectively.

Effective Workout Programming: Designing personalized workout programs, including strength training essentials and advanced techniques for muscle growth.

Cardiovascular Training: Incorporating various cardio methods like HIIT for enhanced endurance and fat loss, complementing strength training routines.

Optimizing Nutrition for Muscle Gain and Fat Loss: Strategies for protein intake, supplements, and dietary approaches tailored to support muscle growth or fat loss goals.

Overcoming Plateaus and Adapting Plans: Adjusting workout intensity, volume, and utilizing psychological strategies to overcome obstacles in fitness progress.

Thank you for embarking on this journey with us. Your commitment to self-improvement and achieving your fitness aspirations is commendable. Here's to your continued success and a healthier, stronger you!